Luminos is the Open Access monograph publishing program
from UC Press. Luminos provides a framework for preserving and
reinvigorating monograph publishing for the future and increases
the reach and visibility of important scholarly work. Titles published
in the UC Press Luminos model are published with the same high
standards for selection, peer review, production, and marketing as
those in our traditional program. www.luminosoa.org

A

BOOK

The Philip E. Lilienthal imprint
honors special books
in commemoration of a man whose work
at University of California Press from 1954 to 1979
was marked by dedication to young authors
and to high standards in the field of Asian Studies.
Friends, family, authors, and foundations have together
endowed the Lilienthal Fund, which enables UC Press
to publish under this imprint selected books
in a way that reflects the taste and judgment
of a great and beloved editor.

The publisher and the University of California Press Foundation
gratefully acknowledge the generous support of the
Philip E. Lilienthal Imprint in Asian Studies, established
by a major gift from Sally Lilienthal.

Making Sense

Making Sense

Language, Ethics, and Understanding in Deaf Nepal

E. Mara Green

UNIVERSITY OF CALIFORNIA PRESS

University of California Press
Oakland, California

© 2024 by E. Mara Green

Suggested citation: Green, E. M., *Making Sense: Language, Ethics, and Understanding in Deaf Nepal*. Oakland: University of California Press, 2024. DOI: https://doi.org/10.1525/luminos.193
Library of Congress Cataloging-in-Publication Data

Names: Green, E. Mara, 1979– author.
Title: Making sense : language, ethics, and understanding in deaf Nepal / E. Mara Green.
Description: Oakland, California : University of California Press, [2024] | Includes bibliographical references and index.
Identifiers: LCCN 2023049682 (print) | LCCN 2023049683 (ebook) | ISBN 9780520399235 (paperback) | ISBN 9780520399242 (ebook)
Subjects: LCSH: Sign language—Social aspects. | Deafness—Social aspects—Nepal. | Deaf—Means of communication—Nepal. | Deaf culture—Nepal. | Deaf—Nepal—Social life and customs.
Classification: LCC HV2471 .G744 2024 (print) | LCC HV2471 (ebook) | DDC 419/.5496—dc23/eng/20240309

LC record available at https://lccn.loc.gov/2023049682
LC ebook record available at https://lccn.loc.gov/2023049683

33 32 31 30 29 28 27 26 25 24
10 9 8 7 6 5 4 3 2 1

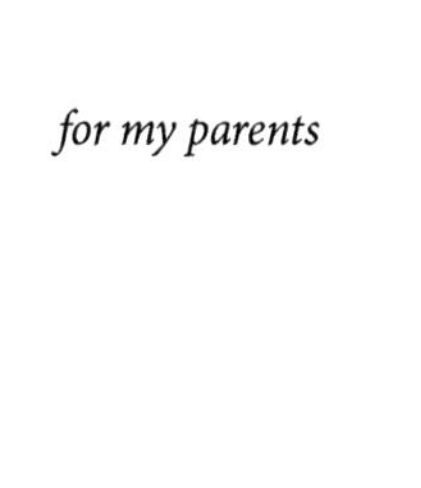

for my parents

CONTENTS

ACKNOWLEDGMENTS

My debts are innumerable, as befits an anthropologist.

I had a vague idea before college that I wanted to study anthropology. At Amherst College, Deborah Gewertz helped me to understand what anthropology could be, and to imagine who I could be as an anthropologist.

In the Anthropology Department at the University of California–Berkeley, William Hanks introduced me to the language of linguistic anthropology. His approach to enduring questions around reference, habit, and presence continues to shape my own. With endless curiosity, Lawrence Cohen so often grasped the best of what I was trying to say or write; I strive to pass this generous gift on to my own students. In Linguistics, Eve Sweetser cultivated space for research on sign and gesture, including their iconic properties, and facilitated the wonderful Berkeley Gesture Group.

Beyond my committee, I am thankful for the courses I took with Saba Mahmood, and for her rigor and humor. Beyond Berkeley, I am grateful for Charles (Chuck) Goodwin's multimodally-oriented work on the ethics of communication, and for his friendship. I wish I could share this book with them. In Anthropology, further thanks are due to Ned Garrett, administrator extraordinaire, and to my friends and classmates, especially James Battle, Himali Dixit, Nathaniel Dumas, Aurora Feeney-Kleinfeldt, Michele Friedner, Andrew Hao, Liz Kelley, Larisa Kurtovic, Xochitl Marsilli-Vargas, Victoria Massey, Eric Plemons, Yancey Orr, Alysoun Quinby, Jade Sasser, Bharat Venkat, and Hallie Wells. In Linguistics, my thanks to Jess Cleary-Kemp (and the rest of her cohort), Andrew Garrett, Sharon Inkelas, Lev Michael, Line Mikkelsen, and Justin Spence, for treating a stray anthropologist as a valued colleague. Katharine Young was the first person to really "see" the importance of my interest in eye gaze. Kate Martineau and Jake Culbertson provided support as I finished the dissertation through an online community facilitated by Alan Klima.

My two years at the University of California–San Diego on a UC President's Postdoctoral Fellowship in the Linguistics Department were a wonderful opportunity to think across fields, and to do so in both English and American Sign Language (ASL). My thanks to Rachel Mayberry, my primary mentor, and Marla Hatrak, lab manager, along with Carol Padden, John Haviland, and Kathryn Woolard for welcoming me into their labs; to Sharon Rose for support on research processes; and to Gabriella Caballero, Sara Goico, Cassandra Hartblay, So-One Hwang, Deniz Ilkbasaran, Ryan Lepic, Amy Lieberman, Hope Morgan, Utpal Sandesara, and Tessa Verhoef for conversations and camaraderie.

My colleagues at Barnard College and Columbia University have been welcoming and supportive from the moment I was hired. Particular thanks to Nadia Abu El-Haj, Vanessa Agard-Jones, Nick Bartlett, Naor Ben-Yehoyada, Brian Boyd, Hannah Chazin, Zoë Crossland, Maria José de Abreu, Catherine Fennell, Severin Fowles, Fabiola Lafontant, Brian Larkin, Elizabeth Povinelli, J.C. Salyer, David Scott, Leslie Sharp, Kaya Williams, and Paige West. To Nick and Naor, thank you for our beautiful, triangular writing group.

This book has been shaped in ways beyond telling by decades-long friendships and exchanges of ideas with Terra Edwards, Michele Friedner, Peter Graif, and Bharat Venkat. I also want to highlight the importance of conversations with John Lee Clark, Lina Hou, Upendra Khanal, Annelies Kusters, Ryan Lepic, Amber Martin, Hope Morgan, Michael Morgan, Erin Moriarty, Angela Nonaka, Rebecca Sanchez, Arjun Shrestha, and Kristin Snoddon.

I thank John Wiley and Sons for permission to use text and images in this book from "The Eye and the Other: Language and Ethics in Deaf Nepal," *American Anthropologist* 124(1):21–38. Terra Edwards, Annelies Kusters, Jack Sidnell, and an anonymous reviewer, along with editors Elizabeth Chin and Deborah Thomas, provided incredibly productive feedback on the article. Elizabeth Chin connected me with artist Nanyi Jiang, who transformed my often-blurry framegrabs into beautiful illustrations for the article and additionally for this book. Working together was such a pleasure, and I am grateful for our collaboration and for her patience across multiple drafts.

The Fulbright Commission, the Social Science Research Council, and the Wenner-Gren Foundation generously funded my dissertation fieldwork, and my applications benefitted from guidance from Bill Hanks, Gillian Hart, and Lev Michael, among others. The Foreign Language and Area Studies program at UC Berkeley, the UC President's Postdoctoral Fellowship, and Barnard College supported additional trips to Nepal. I am also grateful for support from Barnard College, the Wenner-Gren Hunt Fellowship, and the Heyman Center at Columbia University for time dedicated to writing.

I am thankful to have participated in Jane Jones's excellent coaching program, Elevate, where editor Kali Handelman truly got the project. Nick Bartlett, Naor Ben-Yehoyada, Terra Edwards, Michele Friedner, Kristina Jacobsen, Tryphenia Peele, Cate Rhodes, Bharat Venkat, Karen Weingarten, and Hannah Weaver and other members of the Heyman Seminar also read various pieces of the book (sometimes several times) and provided sage advice (only some of which I took). Multiple audiences have also given me useful feedback for which I am grateful.

At the University of California Press, Kate Marshall has been wonderfully supportive of the project and of me. Kristin Snoddon, Marjorie (Candy) Goodwin, Lina Hou, and an anonymous board member offered engaged, generous, and generative readings of my work that helped me to improve the manuscript in key ways. Thank you to Chad Attenborough, Jeff Anderson, Amy Smith Bell, Paige MacKay and Tere Mullin for getting the book, and me, through the production process.

I also want to thank Himali Dixit, Shristi Ghimire, Abinash Pradhan, Bicram Rijal, and Mark Turin for their help with transcribing and translating sometimes-hard-to-hear spoken Nepali. Peter Graif, Muna Gurung, and Dhirendra Nalbo assisted with diacritics and pseudonyms.

This book has multiple beginnings: college, grad school, and my much earlier first experiences signing. I am indebted to Heidi and her mother, whom I met in elementary school and who first taught me sign; and Susie, with whom I first studied ASL at the Deaf Services Bureau in Miami during high school.

And, of course, going to Nepal. I first traveled there in 2002 with the Pitzer in Nepal program: my heartfelt thanks to the staff, my fellow students, and my teachers, and to my host family, the Thapas, and their neighbors, the Pandit Chhetris. During graduate school summers, Sadhana Shrestha and the late Laxminath Shrestha provided tutelage in Nepali, as well as laughter and friendship. Alex von Rospatt helped arrange for me to work with Laxmi-ji and to live with his daughter; Rita-ji and Dristi have become family. My thanks as well to the staff of Fulbright Nepal, in particular Laurie Vasily and Basu Manandhar, and to fellow Fulbrighters Emma Condon, the late Bryan Bushley, Anne Mocko, and especially Miranda Weinberg.

My research, indeed this life as I know it, would not be possible without the welcoming attitude, time, and energy of multiple deaf organizations and countless deaf individuals. My sincere gratitude to the National Federation of the Deaf Nepal, the Kathmandu Association of the Deaf, the Old Deaf Project, the Skill Training Institute for the Deaf, the Gandaki Association of the Deaf, the Dolakha Association of the Deaf, the National Committee of Deaf Women, and deaf schools in several districts. I am especially grateful to the participants of the Old Deaf Project for teaching me so much about communication beyond conventional language.

To my first Nepali Sign Language (NSL) teacher, Kiran Acharya, thank you for welcoming a random hearing American college student into your class. To Uttam Maharjan, Sunita Sherpa, their daughters Manshika and Manshi, and

Rasila Tamang, for being family. My heartfelt gratitude as well to many other deaf and hearing people involved in deaf society: Laxmi Acharya, Sunita Acharya, KP Adhikari, Sunil Ale, Suman Aryal, Kalpana Bajracharya, Kamal Basnet, Bikash Dangol, Parita Dangol, Laxmi Devkota, Tsering Ghale, Anju Ghimire, Bidhya Ghimire, Manju Ghimire, Anju Gurung, Nagendra Gurung, Ranju Hamal, Raghav Bir Joshi, Dinesh KC, Siddhartha KC, Upendra Khanal, Sanu Khimbaja, Rashan Labh, Sangay Lama, Shyam Lama, Sunita Lama, Prasamsa Lamsal, Mahendra Limbu, Laxmi Magar, Anita Maharjan, Dhan Maharjan, Manisha Maharjan, Samundra Nepal, Rajkumar Phuyal, Vivek Rai, Archana Sainju, Suresh Shahi, Pratigya Shakya, Deepak Shakya, Surjan Shakya, Dipawali Sharma, Rajendra Sharma, Shilu Sharma, Chheeri Sherpa, Tsering Sherpa, Chaya Shrestha, Krishna Shrestha, Mohanidevi Shrestha, the late Prasuram Shrestha, the late Ramesh Shrestha, Suraj Shrestha, Tulasi Das Shrestha, Sachin Shrestha, Shreejana Singh, Manish Subba, Dipendra Thapa, Punam Thapa Shrestha, Thulobhai Timilsina, Nirajan Upreti, and Satyadevi Wagle, as well as Bishnu, Gita, Joshi, Karun, Pramila, Roshan, Sabita, Shambhu, Shanti, Sushil, Uday, and individuals who asked me to maintain their anonymity. You helped me to learn NSL and/or natural sign and to orient to the categories, values, and meanings of a world you built together. Many of you also became my friends—thank you. Thank you as well to the students in my English class, who no doubt taught me more than I taught them. Coco Roschaert was a great roommate. In New York City I'm grateful for gatherings with Rabindra Bastola, Laxman Giri, Upendra Khanal, Prasamsa Lamsal, Mohan Panthi, and baby Evani.

Bidhya Ghimire and Shrawan Lal Rai helped get me to Maunabudhuk. I am profoundly grateful to the residents of Maunabudhuk and the neighboring village of Bodhe for their hospitality; to the participants in the 2010 NSL class for allowing me to join in, for sharing the silliest and most serious of conversations, for challenging my vision of what language looks like; to the participants and their families for welcoming me into their homes, video camera and all; and to the class's teacher, whose linguistic, social, and geographical expertise made my work in Maunabudhuk feasible and whose friendship made it a joy.

Particular thanks to Sangita and Arjun Baral, Dewi Basnet, Hira Basnet, Maila Basnet, Purna Maya Basnet, Laxman Bishwakarma, Khadga Bishwakarma, Durga Chemjong, Om Ghimire, Trilochan Giri and his mother, Achyut and Anita Dahal and their daughter Ayusha, Sobha and Indra Khatri and their children and extended families, especially Aryan and Dimpal, Bhim Maya Limbu and her extended family, Dhan Limbu, Dil Kumar Limbu, Harka Maya "Maili" Limbu, Jenisa Limbu, Kanchi Maya Limbu, Man Kumari Limbu, Nil Limbu, Tatu Limbu, Tatu's mom, Bindi Pariyar and her two sons, the late Amrita Pariyar and her mother and sister-in-law, Chandra Tamang, Bhola Thapa, Kamal Yakhha, Matrika *didi* and her husband and children, and many others. Thank you as well to the late Bir Bahadur Shrestha.

I am grateful for the time I spent with Bryan Bushley, Amrita Pariyar, Bir Bahadur Shrestha, Laxminath Shrestha, Prasuram Shrestha, and Ramesh Shrestha.

To all who put their trust in me as a researcher, I hope that my interpretations do, at the very least, make some sense.

Thank you to my former partner, Mindi Sue Spike Shepherd, for her support during graduate school. When she visited me in Nepal, her engagement with signers helped me think about how willingness might be at the heart of the matter.

My extended family (the Green-Minkowski-Minkowsky-Emkin-Seemen-Lindauer network) has been very encouraging of my book-writing endeavors, as have my beloved friends and chosen family, both inside and outside of academia. I am so very grateful to my parents, Steve Green and Karen Minkowski, for the trips we took when my sister and I were little, for encouraging my curiosity, and for unconditional support. Bharat Venkat: I literally would not have finished this book without you.

Finally, to my person, Kelit Brown, for loving me just as I am, for creating a home with me, for understanding me, and—no small feat—for making sure I stay fed and hydrated when I get lost in the writing. You, and we, are so much more than I had ever dared to hope.

In this English-language text I write about multiple communicative practices across several modalities, including Nepali Sign Language (NSL), natural sign/ local sign, and spoken and written Nepali. When I describe these practices, the verb *to sign* is reserved for sign and *to speak* for speech, while verbs like *to say* and *to talk (about)* are used for both.[1]

Sometimes I translate what was said into English, and simply mention how it was said. Other times I draw attention to the form of what was communicated, to its particular existence as a sign, word, concept, or utterance in non-English worlds.

Following academic convention, I represent signs with CAPITAL LETTER GLOSSES. I usually gloss in English but sometimes use Nepali, indicated with *ITALICIZED CAPITAL LETTERS*, as a way of emphasizing the intertwined worlds of Nepali, NSL, and natural sign users.[2]

Words linked by hyphens LIKE-THIS indicate that multiple English words are needed to gloss a single sign. I state explicitly or indicate through context whether glossed signs are NSL or natural/local sign. In some instances I describe a sign's handshape and movement and/or include illustrations.

I use a modified version of the International Alphabet of Sanskrit Transliteration to represent written and spoken Nepali in *italics* followed by a translation 'in single quotes like this.' As per custom, the names of people and places do not include diacritics.

Appendix 4 offers a further guide to transcripts.

Nepali Sign Language (NSL)	English-language name of the signed language used by deaf Nepalis who are part of Nepal's deaf-centered networks or deaf society; NSL has emerged since the founding of Nepal's first permanent school for the deaf in 1966
deaf society	English translation of an NSL phrase (*BAHIRĀ SAMĀJ* 'DEAF SOCIETY') that refers to deaf Nepalis who are involved in deaf schools, organizations, and social networks; NSL is the everyday language of deaf society
natural sign	English translation of an NSL sign (NATURAL-SIGN) that refers to how deaf Nepalis communicate when they do not know NSL, or when they do know NSL but are communicating with deaf or hearing people who do not
local sign	adaptation of a mixed English-Nepali phrase used by hearing Nepali speakers in Maunabudhuk, in eastern Nepal, to differentiate between local signing practices (which NSL signers would refer to as natural sign) and NSL
conventional language	language as most people experience and think about it, in which shared grammar does a great deal of unnoticed work; examples include Nepali Sign Language, Nepali, American Sign Language, and English

emergent language — communicative practices that depend as much on shared desire to communicate as on shared grammar; emergent language requires heightened labor and attention; examples include natural/local sign in Nepal, less conventionalized instances of International Sign, and some instances of communication by/with people with disabilities such as aphasia

communicative sociality — the dimension of being (in relation) with others that involves talking with them in any modality

communicative or interactional vulnerability — heightened possibility of being ignored, misunderstood, or not-understood due to context-specific communicative asymmetries

Introduction

One day in June 2010 in Maunabudhuk, a village in eastern Nepal, Shrila Khadka, a fifty-year-old deaf woman, signed to a younger hearing woman as they stood in a tea shop, surrounded by wooden tables and water pitchers. Speaking Nepali, the hearing woman said that she didn't understand. Meanwhile, her gaze slid away from Shrila's hands and face. A second young hearing woman present exclaimed in spoken Nepali, "She said you should come to her house and her daughter-in-law will make you tea. Don't you even understand that much?"[1] Despite the woman's scolding words, and despite the profound ordinariness of the setting and topic, it was by no means a given that a hearing person, or for that matter another deaf person, would understand Shrila's invitation.

This scene points to and challenges two entwined assumptions about human sociality that are so foundational in the social sciences and in many people's everyday lives that they tend to go unstated. The first is that to be human is to be born into a world of accessible language. Deaf studies, sign language linguistics, and allied fields have disproven this supposition by documenting the experiences of deaf people, the vast majority of whom are born into hearing, nonsigning families. Indeed, for many such deaf people, learning a conventional signed language and becoming part of a deaf community or communities is a transformative process (Padden and Humphries 1988; Ladd 2003; Monaghan et al. 2003; Bechter 2008; Friedner 2014; Kraus 2018).[2] The second, corollary assumption is that in everyday life, people can count on their own and others' intelligibility. Nearly all studies on "deaf sociality" (Friedner 2015) and communicative practices— including this one—challenge the factuality of this assumption *and* underscore that signing environments matter because they enable deaf people to experience the ease of shared language, of understanding and being understood (Mathur and Napoli 2011; Friedner 2016). This idea is critical in work on nationally scaled deaf communities as well as in places known as "shared signing communities" (Kisch 2008), characterized by high percentages of deaf people and widespread use of a signed language.

But Shrila's circumstances are distinct both from those of people raised in robust signing environments and those of people who encounter such environments later in life. She communicates in what, following users of Nepali Sign Language (NSL), I call *natural sign*. (Throughout this book I draw on the terminology and concepts of NSL signers a great deal.) Briefly put, natural sign involves a small repertoire of widely available, shared signs complemented by strategies that make use of the body's capacity to point to and mimetically represent places, people, movements, objects, and other elements of the social world. Natural sign practices vary but are more conventional and conventionally understood across signers than *home sign*, and less so than *shared sign languages* and *emerging sign languages*—three key categories in the literature (discussed more in chapter 2). Across persons and contexts, natural signers experience a range of responses from those with whom they try to communicate—from not-understanding to understanding, as the vignette with Shrila demonstrates. This unevenness is a pervasive and consequential characteristic of natural sign conversations. I witnessed lively natural sign conversations about politics, love, yesterday's gossip, or tomorrow's work plans, on the one hand, and conversations that came to a grinding halt, or failed to occur in the first place, on the other. The immense variability in whether, what, and how people communicate and understand is one of natural sign's most socially significant and intellectually puzzling characteristics. The contradiction that animates this book is the fact that in natural sign, referential understanding is possible yet precarious, often achieved but never guaranteed.[3]

All language users experience the possibility of being misunderstood, not-understood, or even ignored. Yet most language users, at least in specific circumstances, get to take for granted that they will understand and be understood "well enough" for the purposes at hand—and that if not, a change in who they are talking with, or what language, dialect, or modality is in use, will yield the sought-after understanding.[4] But for Shrila, there is no otherwise; having someone to whom she was signing directly not understand her was par for the course. Grounded in long-term fieldwork with deaf and hearing people in Nepal, this book explores what it means to communicate when understanding and being understood are radically contingent and persistently in question.

It is tempting to analyze the discrepancy between how the two hearing women responded to Shrila by positing a difference in how well they "know" natural sign. Hearing people in Maunabudhuk and the adjacent village of Bodhe have a range of relationships to deaf people and signing. Deaf people live throughout the area, constituting roughly 1 percent of the total population; some hearing people grow up with deaf family members or close neighbors, while others interact with deaf people far less frequently. Any given individual, deaf or hearing, thus has more or less exposure to and experience with producing and seeing others produce sign.

And familiarity with natural sign certainly matters. I learned this through communicating in natural sign as well as watching others do so. Prior to conducting fieldwork in Maunabudhuk, I had gained some practice communicating in natural sign in Kathmandu, spending time at a program for elderly deaf people. When I moved to Maunabudhuk, I was able to draw on some particular signs I had acquired as well as general strategies for communicating in natural sign. I also learned signs that I had not encountered in Kathmandu, simultaneously becoming familiar with the broader social and material context. For example, many people in Maunabudhuk raise pigs. I learned how pigs are butchered, with a sharp stab to the chest, that PIG is signed with an index finger jabbed into the signer's own ribs, that eating pork is associated with certain ethnic groups, and that asking "PIG EAT?" is one way of ascertaining ethnicity. For people who grew up in the area, these visual, kinetic, cognitive, and social associations are part of what makes natural sign usage possible. While the degree of conventionality in natural sign is limited when compared to languages like Nepali Sign Language, American Sign Language, Nepali, or English, there are conventional natural signs in domains as varied as kinship, places and events, and agricultural and household activities. There are also some conventions in the way that signs get combined.

If, however, "knowing" natural sign were all that mattered, variability in people's responses to natural sign conversations would be no more puzzling than the fact that some people know NSL or Nepali and some people do not. Critically, many natural signs, whether conventional or improvised in the course of conversation, involve potentially "decipherable" (Kuschel 1973) relationships between form and meaning—as suggested by PIG. Natural sign offers the possibility that someone might figure out the articulation and meaning of a new-to-them sign. I analyze these signs as *immanent* in the sociomaterial context. Put another way, the relationship between the signed modality and the world itself offers communicative potential. For example, signers can point at and thus direct addressees' attention to objects, people, and places. I learned that a village visible across a valley was named Kurule and that many women who had married into families in Maunabudhuk had grown up there. For these women, pointing toward Kurule could invoke their birth family or the time period of childhood.

Signers also use their bodies to indicate actions, sizes, shapes, and qualities that addressees can (try to) recognize and connect with social patterns. For example, people in farming communities know that cornfields should be weeded when the corn plants reach a certain height; that knowledge is available for representation through the body by means of using a hand to indicate height—and thus by extension, the time when that happens. Similarly, in Maunabudhuk and Bodhe, stone grinders adorn many porches; a signer who moves one fist in a horizontal circle can evoke an understanding of grinding flour because the addressee has seen or performed this movement even if she has never seen or done it qua linguistic sign.

As another example, *bhāi ṭikā din* is a ritual and holiday celebrated by many Nepalis during a series of holidays known collectively as Tihar. *Ṭikā* is a ceremonial powder or paste placed on foreheads during celebrations; *bhāi ṭikā din* means 'younger brother's *ṭikā* day' and focuses on the relationship between brothers and sisters. On this day, families tend to dress up. Gifts of money or cloth are given or received, as are sweets. Food is consumed. But these are actions also typical of other holidays and rituals. In contrast, it is only during *bhāi ṭikā din* that siblings carefully place colored dots of *ṭikā* in vertical lines on each other's foreheads; moreover, *bhāi ṭikā din* is for many the pinnacle event during Tihar. Signers refer to *bhāi ṭikā din* and to Tihar more generally by using their fingers to enact the placing of those dots, or to point to the location of those dots, albeit on the signer's own forehead. The sign is immanent in the social practice and structure of the holiday; the world nudges signers to refer to Tihar in this way. Immanence means that communication beyond (or before) conventionality is quite possible, in a way that does not seem to be available in speech/sound. Building on a long tradition in sign language studies of thinking about how the signed modality offers affordances for iconic and indexical representation (Kuschel 1973; Kendon 1980b; Taub 2001; Liddell 2003; Dudis 2004, 2011; Cuxac and Sallandre 2008; Padden et al. 2013, 2105), I emphasize here how the sociomaterial world of bodies, landscapes, and routines in which signs are produced and interpreted offers itself up for use in the production and interpretation of those signs.[5]

The demographic and semiotic characteristics of natural sign are necessary for explaining variability in what communication in natural sign looks like, and why understanding is so uneven, as with Shrila's interlocutors. But accounting for natural sign in these terms is not enough. Returning to the opening vignette, recall that the first woman, even as she said that she could not understand, stopped looking at Shrila. Looking away from a signer is a particularly obvious way for a potential addressee to both signal a disinterest in, and enact a barrier to, understanding. The vignette demonstrates quite literally that to understand natural sign, addressees must be willing to look. Even if the woman had continued to look at Shrila, however, she might have been uninvested in trying to understand and put together the meanings of the signs—in trying to *make sense* of what Shrila had said. Addressees, in other words, must be willing to try.

This ethnographic argument recursively underpins the book's primary methodological and theoretical argument. Interactionally, making sense in natural sign requires that interlocutors attend to each other and try to understand each other; methodologically and theoretically, making sense of natural sign requires that I attend to social and semiotic relations, and to the willingness, or unwillingness, of potential interlocutors to do the work of communicating. I approach willingness, unwillingness, and a range of other embodied orientations through the framework of ethics, which emphasizes both the depth and nuance of the entanglement of selves with others (and others with selves) as well as the sometimes unpredictable, sometimes unintended, but nevertheless pervasively consequential effects of people's actions on others.

Natural sign, as a communicative practice, both highlights and heightens the ethical foundations of all language. Chatting about existential dilemmas in a language a person has known since before memory, politely trying to purchase fruit in a language they are just learning, reading dense academic texts, or commenting casually on social media posts: linguistic communication involves work, whether framed as cognitive, embodied, or interpretive. It involves a turning-toward, a desire, an orientation (Weber 1947; Hanks 1996; Goodwin 2006; Green 2014a, 2022a; Friedner 2015). Refusal or unwillingness to engage in sense-making is its own kind of orienting, a turning-away.[6]

Thus natural sign lays bare the bones of human communication: the way others must attend to someone in order for them to be understood; the way that making sense *to* someone requires that they make sense *of* you; the entanglement of word with world, language with context, semiotics with sociality. Natural sign shows that ethics is not only intrinsic to linguistic interaction but also grounds its very possibility. While ultimately true for all language use, natural sign heightens this relationship and its consequences, in terms of both interaction (how and whether people understand) and analysis (how scholars understand whether people understand). The particularities of natural sign demand something more and perhaps different from potential interlocutors than conversation in conventional language: more attention, more labor, more willingness. Drawing on lean conventionality and semiotic immanence, natural signers can and do use various resources in skillful and creative ways (Green 2017, 2022b). Both expressing and understanding what gets said, however, requires people to do more work than they do with conventional languages. While all communication requires that addressees make inferences about "what is meant" beyond "what is said," interlocutors using natural sign must, to varying degrees, also do the work to infer what is being said.[7] Such work is not guaranteed. People may, and often do, choose not to engage. They may also try to engage and nevertheless fail to understand or be understood. Or they may understand, as the second hearing woman understood Shrila.

Throughout this book my goal is to center deaf signers as creative and expert communicators and theorists. This goal draws on and responds to anthropological traditions of grounding analysis in local categories and concepts (e.g., Mahmood 2001); growing calls from deaf scholars to center deaf epistemologies and ontologies (e.g., Kusters, De Meulder, and O'Brien 2017); and research in linguistics that troubles the often implicit hierarchy of academic over lay and Western over non-Western approaches to language (e.g., Hanks, Ide, and Katagiri 2009; Kusters and Sahasrabudhe 2018).[8] As chapter 1 explores in detail, NSL signers both cherish NSL—itself a marginalized language—and recognize that natural sign enables them to communicate with non-NSL signers, both deaf and hearing.[9] Most deaf Nepalis, in fact, use natural sign as their primary communicative mode, sometimes alongside some use of one of Nepal's many spoken languages. Natural sign does not involve a lot of metalinguistic talk; but NSL discourse is replete with it, and NSL signers have much to say about natural sign—in fact, they posit the very existence of the category. I move between thinking and writing about natural sign as a metalinguistic category and natural sign as an interactional phenomenon. In terms of the latter, most of my data is from Maunabudhuk and the adjacent village of Bodhe, where Nepali speakers sometimes distinguished between NSL and, using the English word, "local" sign.[10] I use *natural sign* and *local sign* as overlapping though not exactly equivalent metalinguistic terms; the former refers to this mode of signing throughout Nepal, including in Maunabudhuk and Bodhe, whereas the latter is reserved specifically for these two villages.[11]

LANGUAGE, BODIES, AND MATERIALITY IN SOCIAL THEORY

In anthropology and related fields, it has become fashionable to dismiss scholarship that focuses on the referential or propositional functions of language: how people use language to create shared understandings on the level of what heuristically can be called content. Such dismissals often invoke Saussure's (1972) model of the talking heads (figure 1), but only to point out how much it oversimplifies, as indeed it does.

Language is not only oral and aural. Language can be produced and received in the visual signed modality (Stokoe 1960; Klima and Bellugi 1979; Padden and Perlmutter 1987) and the tactile modality (granda and Nuccio 2018; Edwards and Brentari 2020; Clark and Nuccio 2020). Some language users communicate primarily or only through written/typed text (Sequenzia and Grace 2015). Moreover, alternative theories of semiotics such as Peirce's (1955), and younger disciplines like neurolinguistics, show that language does not neatly transfer from one person's mind to another's via sensory input. Understanding what someone else has meant involves complex neurological, psychological, and social processes. But to entirely dismiss the talking heads model is to disregard what it gets right, or at least what it captures about many people's experience: on the level of reference, in everyday conversations, people often understand each other quite well. When you say, "I hate lima beans," I know you mean *lima beans*, not *kidney beans*, and if I mistake one for the other, my mistake can be identified and probably corrected. And I know you mean you strongly dislike them, not that you are allergic to them (though you might use the phrase "allergic to" more loosely, to mean you hate them a lot).

My broader point here is that despite claims to the contrary, signifier and signified have not come apart. If they had, neither that sentence nor this one could have

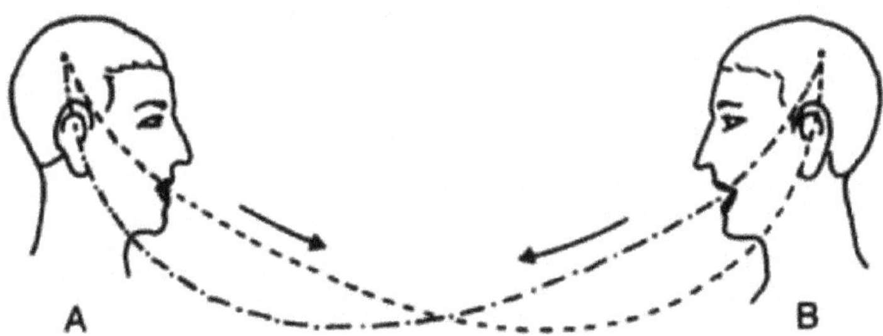

FIGURE 1. Saussure's talking heads (1972:11): a drawing of two heads facing each other, labeled A and B. One line moves from A's upper head to A's mouth to B's ear to B's upper head. A second line traces the reverse trajectory, from B's head to B's mouth to A's ear to A's head. Reproduced by permission from Open Court, a division of Cricket Media.

been written or understood. Indeed the functions of language (Jakobson 1960) that are not (only) referential almost always depend on referentiality—I include here referentiality that is mediated by interpreters and translators—and critiques of referentiality depend on reference to be understood in the first place. There are important exceptions; patients *not* understanding shamanic healing rituals may in fact be at the heart of such rituals' efficacy (Briggs 1996; Hanks 2012), and the "denotational unintelligibility" of glossolalia produces important social and devotional effects (Harkness 2017). In both cases, however, it is assumed that what is being said makes sense to *someone*—the shaman, the ancestors, the gods, or God—and this presumed intelligibility is critical to the power of the ritual or prayer.

The important attention paid to the many ways that human language use is more than referential often takes reference for granted. And in fact most people *can* take it for granted, at least most of the time. But not everyone; Shrila certainly can't. This book thus asks what happens to people's experiences of language and sociality, as well as to foundational social scientific accounts of those experiences, when referentiality itself is in question. What are the experiential, ethical, and intellectual stakes of living in and thinking with worlds wherein language cannot be taken for granted?

To begin to answer these questions, it is critical to interrogate what assumptions about bodies, minds, and senses are woven into how social scientists theorize and make claims. Take, for example, a primal scene in the social scientific imagination: Althusser's 1971 example of interpellation. He asks the reader to imagine a scene of "the most commonplace everyday police (or other) hailing": "There are individuals walking along. Somewhere (usually behind them) the hail rings out: 'Hey, you there!' One individual (nine times out of ten it is the right one) turns round, believing/suspecting/knowing that it is for him, i.e. recognizing that 'it really is he' who is meant by the hailing" (1971:174–175). Althusser is careful to note that "in reality these things happen without any succession" (1971:172); the scene is supposed to be read as metaphorical, or at least, as not exactly real. But, as Kunreuther (2014:10, emphasis added) argues in her analysis of voice, Althusser is specifically theorizing how "an individual becomes a subject, endowed with consciousness, desires, and specific values, through *reiterated forms of address and conventions* that delineate a social position." In other words, the metaphor is also the actual means of subject-making. Building on Kunreuther, I argue that it is necessary to take seriously the scene's material and communicative dimensions more broadly. Althusser assumes that the "individuals walking along," as well as the police, are speakers and hearers, not just in Goffman's (1981) sense of participating in a communicative relationship but also in bodily terms.

Both the call, "Hey, you there," and the response, turning around upon recognizing that the call is meant for oneself, require bodies that literally speak and hear. I first wrote about this scene in relation to deaf people in 2013 or 2014, and it was only in 2021 that I really noticed the phrase "walking along." The naturalization of certain kinds of bodies is endless. The fact that the call comes from behind further effaces modality and the senses, in that if the sound of speech is enough to draw attention to the fact that someone is speaking, people must have been able to hear it. Moreover, the individual who recognizes themself as hailed seems not only to have heard the police's call but also to have understood it—and this seems to be true as well for the other people, those not hailed directly, whom Goffman would call overhearers. With this seamless hailing and response exemplifying the process of interpellation, social actors or subjects are naturalized as having normatively configured minds and bodies and as sharing a conventional, spoken language.[12]

Of course language is not the only way people are interpellated. The cry "It's a boy/girl!" indexes and instantiates an entire apparatus of linguistic and non-linguistic ways that people are gendered (Butler 1997). Senghas (2003:271–272) argues that deaf Nicaraguans who are "linguistically isolated" from their hearing compatriots are unmistakably Nicaraguan. People turn when called, or run away in terror, as much because of the institutional force of the police as because of language—and this is in fact part of Althusser's point.[13] I am not claiming that social and political systems do not hail and interpellate deaf people. Rather, I am arguing for careful attention to unstated and therefore unnoticed assumptions about the actual means through which interpellation, subjectification, and other foundational social processes happen. I am arguing that in both theory and everyday life, the linguistic and material modes through which persons come into relation with one another matter.

Language draws people in through the sensory capacities of bodies, the material affordances of sound, sight, and touch, and the force of shared grammar, or at least a shared understanding of what language sounds, looks, or feels like. What happens when this sharedness cannot be taken for granted? As in the opening vignette, on multiple occasions I saw hearing people look or wander away from deaf people who were signing to them. People seem to feel able to ignore what has been said when they do not understand it. How might natural sign—not fully shared, not fully conventional—unhook hearing, and occasionally other deaf, people from the responsibility to be socially hailed, not so much by the police as by deaf relatives, friends, and neighbors? And how do the ethical foundations of communication become literally visible in such cases?

LANGUAGE AND ORDINARY ETHICS

An important recent focus of scholarship on ethical practice in everyday life centers on how people act in relation to others and how the substance, contours, and actions of the self are shaped by the presence and particularity of those others (Lambek ed. 2010; Pandian and Ali 2010; Faubion 2011; Das 2012; Venkat 2017). Sometimes referred to as *ordinary ethics*, these approaches do not set out to draw a sharp line between the ordinary and nonordinary—after all, what is ordinary is historically, culturally, and biographically contingent—but rather to call attention both to the capaciousness of ethical orientations, actions, and consequences in social life and to the usefulness of ethics as an analytic (Lambek 2010). Following Lambek (2010:8–9), I am not invested in distinguishing between morality and ethics, and I use the category of the ethical in "the broader sense," such that it includes what from other perspectives might be labeled unethical actions or consequences.

Ordinary ethical actions are routinely incorporated into the bodily practices of life with others and nevertheless performed with purpose and care (Das 2012:135). This duality characterizes much of ordinary ethical action (Lambek 2010). In the settings I write about, orienting to a signer or not is both habitual and agentive, located in the space between what Lambek (2010:6), citing a much "old[er] distinction," refers to as the "is" and the "ought." Drawing on Keane (2016), it might be said that routine tasks and interactions offer ethical affordances or opportunities for ethical expression. As Das (2012) describes: How do you make tea for each member of your family? When your partner comes home at the end of a workday, how do you greet them? These "minutest of gestures" (Das 2012:135) are in the case of natural sign quite literal: the making of signs, the direction of eye gaze. Ordinary ethical practices can also include the everyday actions of people who seek to transform the world such that it is more fully inhabitable by marginalized groups such as deaf or queer people (Dave 2012; Friedner 2015). There are important resonances between these kinds of ethical projects and the ones taken on by NSL signers that I explore in chapter 1. NSL signers' efforts to learn NSL, to become members of *BAHIRĀ SAMĀJ* 'DEAF SOCIETY,' to teach others NSL, and to cultivate an ever-larger deaf society are acts both of self- and world-making.[14]

NSL signers understand themselves as responsible for other deaf people in fairly expansive ways; they also talk about hearing people's responsibilities. Sagar Karki, a deaf NSL teacher with whom I worked closely, once told an audience of hearing people that shopkeepers have a duty to talk in turn with deaf and hearing customers.[15] He was not suggesting that all shopkeepers, let alone all hearing people, could or even should learn NSL but rather that shopkeepers, and hearing people more broadly, could communicate with deaf people in natural sign *if they bothered to do so.* I understand this less as a call for building a radically different world and more as a call for attending to and actualizing a world that already can or even does exist; my attention to such a call is thus as much an anthropology of the *meanwhile* as it is an anthropology of the *otherwise* (Povinelli 2011).[16] Sagar's call also highlights how a social actor, such as a hearing shopkeeper, might or might not understand their own practices as ethical in nature, while still having profound ethical consequences. Forgetting that someone likes clotted milk in their tea may result in hurt feelings. Forgetting that over and over again may result in a rift in a relationship. Not engaging with someone's signing results in a rift in not just a relationship but relationality itself.

Sagar's admonishment that shopkeepers should interact with both deaf and hearing people, rather than shoo away deaf customers, resonates with the anthropological assertion that interaction is an inherently ethical domain (Garfinkel 1963, 1967, cited in Heritage 1984; Goodwin 2006; Sidnell 2010; Keane 2016; Green 2022a). Interaction requires that people establish and maintain relations through corporeal and cognitive acts of attention and turn-taking (Goffman 1964, 1967, cited in Goffman 1981; Duranti and Goodwin 1992:148; Sidnell 2010). And both the person talking and their addressees must do further work, on several levels. Not everything "talked about" is explicitly "mentioned" (Garfinkel 1963:221, cited in Heritage 1984:81). Hanks (1990) shows that even reference is a socially complex endeavor, while Kockelman (2005:245) proposes that "pragmatics is prior to semantics." Put another way, even what *does* get explicitly mentioned does not simply make sense; someone must make sense of it (De Jaegher and Di Paolo 2007). Addressees must figure out what is meant from multiple "possible interpretations" (D. Cameron 1998:439), and interlocutors have a "moral" expectation of each other to do "whatever is necessary" to understand (Heritage 1984:82, 95). This relies on the addressee's "commitment" and "degree of *hermeneutic openness*" (Kockelman 2005:251–252, 261, italics in original).[17]

Yet the claim that speakers/signers and addressees do work, including at the level of semantics and reference, is in tension with how most people experience language and understanding—as "automatic and obligate" to use Levinson's words (2006:52), illustrated earlier by my discussion of Althusser. I draw on Hanks (1990) and Rumsey (2010) to resolve this tension. Hanks utilizes the concept of *habitus* to explain how linguistic structures get reproduced in novel utterances; grammar is the sedimentation of habit, and particular instances of habitual language use (re)animate grammar. Rumsey (2010:206), meanwhile, argues that ethical action "is not only enabled by language but is positively required by it": when people speak or sign, they cannot help but inhabit ethical positions, such as an *I* in relation to a *you*, that are grammatically encoded by language. Bringing these approaches together, I argue that grammar performs not only cognitive and communicative but also ethical labor for its users (Green 2022a). Each time someone understands someone else without effort, or despite being distracted, bored, indifferent, or even hostile, grammar is doing powerful but unnoticed work for both the person talking and the addressee. By hooking people into a robust grammatical system that facilitates easeful communication, conventional language does a great deal to let its users off the hook in ethical terms.[18]

If conventional language provides ethical scaffolds, it is unsurprising that emergent language practices offer especially generative material for thinking about the ethical underpinnings and processes of communication. Here it is helpful to expand on the distinction between conventional language and emergent language that I introduced in the preliminary definitions. *Conventional language* refers to language as most people in the world experience and think about it. Conversing with others who share your language, whether spoken or signed, is an instance of conventional language. Processing it is experienced as "immediate and obligate," to return to Levinson's phrase. *Emergent language*, of which natural sign is one mode, involves more putting-together, more work, more guessing, more back-and-forth. Conventional language in use also has emergent properties, and emergent language makes use of conventions, whether linguistic or otherwise. These are heuristic categories, the purpose being to draw attention to the qualities of emergence and conventionality as they manifest in particular settings, and to aid in analyzing the social consequences of those qualities.[19]

Emergent language practices, whether classified as signing or not, often involve modes of meaning-making such as pointing, gesture, or object incorporation, that offer some kind of possibility for decipherability (e.g., Goodwin 2006; Levinson 2006; Kusters dir. 2015). But this possibility—as opposed to the more immediate understanding produced by conventional language—means that it is critical that people *want* to make sense of each other. Goodwin (2006), for example, writes about his father, who had aphasia following a stroke and communicated primarily with gestures, prosody, and several English words. Goodwin (2006:106) explicitly states that his father's conversational partners, who work with him to produce meaningful utterances, consider him "someone who is trying to say something relevant"—an orientation that is fundamentally "moral" in nature.[20]

I also build on prior work that theorizes signing as moral practice. Nonaka (2007:15) suggests that in shared signing communities such as Ban Khor, Thailand, a shared language and what she calls a "moral habitus" of use (which includes "the willingness of hearing people to acquire and use that language") coemerge over time. In what is broadly known as International Sign (IS), signers consider communication across different signed languages to be not only possible but also morally valuable (Green 2014c).[21] Friedner (2015) documents how new and experienced Indian Sign Language (ISL) signers frequently check in with each other about their understanding and repeat information for each other, characterizing deaf, ISL-centered spaces as "moral." But the case of natural sign is distinct from these examples. Unlike Ban Khor, the settings where I have researched natural sign do not have familial and geographical social clusters in which signing, and orienting to it, have become fully habitual for some critical number of people, both deaf and hearing. Unlike in the kinds of international encounters where signers use International Sign, not everyone has another language to fall back on, nor is there a shared commitment to mutual moral orientation. And unlike in urban deaf India, these are mixed deaf-hearing spaces, lacking the kind of moral imperative to create deaf similitude and to orient toward collective understanding and "deaf development" (Friedner 2015).

In writing about natural sign and natural signers in Nepal, I bring together an ethical perspective on language and interaction with an ever-growing body of research on deaf communication, and in particular the communication of deaf people who are not part of deaf communities or shared signing communities (at least as classically defined), or who are but are communicating with hearing people (e.g., Kuschel 1973; Kendon 1980a, 1980b, 1980c; Goldin-Meadow et al. 1984; Jepson 1991a, 1991b; Torigoe, Takei, and Kimura 1995; Torigoe and Takei 2002; Fox Tree 2009, 2011; Haviland 2013; Kusters dir. 2015; Hou 2016, 2020; Kusters 2017, 2019; Kusters and Sahasrabudhe 2018; Reed et al. 2018; Moriarty 2019; Goico 2019; Horton 2020a, 2020b; Neveu 2020; Reed 2022; Friedner 2022). I argue that communication in emergent language is not only influenced by and reflective of its sociocultural contexts, it is literally made possible or impossible by them. When the forms and structures of conventional language are not in reach, language users—signers/speakers and addressees—are asked to pick up the slack; sometimes they do, and sometimes they don't; sometimes they succeed, and sometimes they don't. In natural sign, questions of bodily and cognitive attention, nonlinguistic knowledge shared or unshared by interlocutors, and interlocutors' desire and willingness, become more perceptible, salient, and consequential than in conventional language use. Indeed, I argue, the processes of semiotic interpretation and ethical orientation become indistinguishable in certain moments.

Natural signers' participation in everyday modes of *communicative sociality* is therefore profoundly vulnerable to ordinary ethical actions, such as averting one's gaze, as in the opening vignette in this introduction. Moreover, potential interlocutors' orientations toward communicating with natural signers can render them (un)intelligible, not only in the moment but as persons more generally. This is evident in the commonly-used spoken Nepali word *lāṭo*, which connotes someone who doesn't make sense and is colloquially used to refer to deaf people—a word that NSL signers abhor and that they critique from the position of keen awareness of their vulnerability when using natural sign with hearing interlocutors.

There are times when being misunderstood or not-understood has self-evidently high stakes, and not only for natural signers. In a devastating passage, Goodwin (2006:106) writes about how his father's catheter was inserted incorrectly following a stroke, but the doctors "dismissed" as meaningless his gestures and speech when he tried to tell them so. In Nepal, I recall discussing with women NSL signers the particularly painful situation faced by deaf girls and women who had been raped and who were not NSL signers and thus were not understood or believed when they tried to describe or identify their attacker.[22] Deaf elders at the Old Deaf Project in Kathmandu told stories about being cheated out of land by unscrupulous hearing siblings, illustrating how deaf people's material disempowerment, especially that of natural signers, is linked to language and communication.

There are important moments in this book that concern memories and allegations of mistreatment and violence. Recognizing with Das (2007) that violence can be ordinary and everyday, I nevertheless want to emphasize that many of the situations I write about are quite mundane: whether someone is understood when she makes casual conversation at a communal water tap; how someone else is evaluated when misunderstandings arise about how long she was out of town; what it takes for a signer to secure someone's interest in chatting. I argue that it is precisely this everydayness that makes the stakes of understanding and being understood different for natural signers than for users of conventional but marginalized languages, whether signed or spoken.

When NSL signers are misunderstood or treated poorly by hearing people— whether they are using natural sign, NSL, writing, speech, or some combination —they have both behind and ahead of them experiences of linguistic ease and more or less consistent mutual understanding with other NSL signers. Natural signers, especially those who struggle the most with everyday communication (chapter 5), have no such horizon. NSL signers can chart specific moments when their (hearing) interlocutors ignore them, fail to understand, or misunderstand, against the memory and expectation of shared intelligibility. For deaf natural signers the juxtaposition of willingness and refusal, of understanding, misunderstanding, and not-understanding, of being attended to and ignored, saturates the ordinary. The horizons of yesterday and tomorrow look just like right here, right now. It is this profound ordinariness that makes the stakes of thinking with and through natural sign so high.

HOW I CAME TO WRITE THIS BOOK

I first spent time in Nepal in 2002, as a hearing undergraduate student on a study abroad program focused on cultural immersion and learning spoken Nepali. At that time, I was a decent American Sign Language (ASL) signer and was interested in meeting deaf signers in Nepal. My program connected me to the Kathmandu Association of the Deaf (KAD), where I was greeted warmly by deaf members and board members as well as hearing interpreters. Over the next three weeks a deaf teacher at KAD generously allowed me to sit in on his NSL class, and deaf interlocutors showed me around Nepal's oldest deaf residential school, invited me into their homes and to a wedding feast, and took me to the Bakery Café, which employed a large number of deaf staff, and to the Skill Training Institute for the Deaf (STID), where I met young women who had only recently begun to learn NSL. I remember at least one deaf interlocutor telling me emphatically how different deaf people's experiences are "in the villages." (As I relate in chapter 1, I learned later that "the village" is shorthand for places without networks of NSL signers.) These experiences sparked my interest in deaf Nepalis who are not NSL signers.

I returned to Nepal in the summers of 2006 and 2008 as a graduate student in anthropology and conducted my dissertation fieldwork, which forms the core of this book, from September 2009 to December 2010. I knew by then that I wanted to engage with people whom I now call natural signers by embedding myself in an NSL outreach program run by the National Federation of the Deaf Nepal (abbreviated NDFN to distinguish it from the National Federation of the Disabled Nepal, NFDN). One cycle of classes was ending when I arrived in the fall of 2009. Among several locations in spring 2010, Maunabudhuk in Dhankuta district seemed like a good fit. The NDFN generously agreed to my request to do research and helped facilitate my arrival in Maunabudhuk several weeks into the six-month program. There I met the deaf teacher, as well as the deaf participants from both Maunabudhuk and the adjoining village of Bodhe. One teenager attended briefly; the other participants were adults in their thirties to sixties. Ten of them attended regularly, and three others more sporadically. I lived in Maunabudhuk from the end of April through the end of October of 2010.

My goal was not to study the NSL class per se, but the class certainly had effects both on the process of research and on the everyday lives and communicative practices of deaf villagers and their hearing interlocutors. The class gathered deaf residents regularly in a way that had not occurred prior. Moreover, NSL teacher Sagar Karki's pedagogical goals and my research goals happily coincided; we both, for example, wanted to spend time visiting the homes of the deaf people who participated in the class. His linguistic and social expertise became critical to my research process; he in turn expressed how glad he was to have the company of an NSL signer during the long afternoon hours after the morning class. My daily presence in class, and the fact that Sagar and I frequently visited deaf people's homes together, also worked to position me in particular ways. As discussed in the following chapter, Sagar seemed to disturb hearing people's sense of the category *deaf*. In contrast, I seemed to fit relatively well into the category of a hearing, white, foreign/American *mis* 'miss, teacher,' familiar from United States Peace Corps Volunteers who had worked in the village.[23]

And in fact, there were many times when I did take up a teaching role. Hearing teenagers and adults who stopped by the class even momentarily would frequently take up a teaching role during literacy instruction; for me to refrain from helping deaf students with their letters or the NSL signs that I knew would have been considered odd and selfish. The NSL class was a source of value for participants but also of friction (Green 2014c), as attendance meant that they couldn't perform household and farm labor during class and while they walked to and from their homes. Several deaf people asked Sagar and me to intervene with their families, suggesting that they were being asked to bear too great a workload in comparison to their hearing family members and/or to miss class too frequently. Such requests for intervention were one of the ways that I was positioned as being an advocate for deaf people in addition to being a researcher.

When hearing people verbalized an assumption that I was a teacher or even the one in charge of the NSL program, however, I would reply that I wasn't in actuality a *mis* 'teacher,' that I was there to conduct fieldwork, that Sagar was the teacher. I did so not only to inform or remind people of my research purposes but also because I desperately wanted to make it clear that deaf people are teachers too and that the respect due to educators should be directed toward Sagar. More generally, while being (regarded as) a teacher made me legible to Maunabudhuk's residents, it also often felt at odds with my role as researcher and learner—of local communicative practices, relationships, geography. I was (almost) always glad therefore when my incompetence was revealed, as when I got lost on pathways (happily reported by Sagar to his students), spilled water on myself when attempting to drink water with the appropriate gap between my mouth and the vessel, or naively wondered what a human-made hole in the ground was for (sewage!). It is also worth noting that along with "Mara *mis*," I was addressed and referred to with the phrases "Mara *bahini* 'younger sister,'" "Mara *didi* 'older sister,'" and "Mara *anṭi* 'auntie.'"

I returned to Kathmandu and Maunabudhuk during summer trips in 2012, 2015, and 2018. I had been hoping to spend time there again during 2020 or 2021, but the universe has had different plans. Across nearly two years of fieldwork, in addition to spending time at deaf organizations, classes, and conferences, I have spent time with friends and acquaintances celebrating New Year, Holi, Tihar, and other holidays, learning how to properly cook *chiyā* 'tea,' attending soccer matches and cricket practice, discussing the intricacies of organizational politics, arguing about which bus to take, wandering through Kathmandu's crowded streets in search of the perfect jacket, exchanging stories of childhood and love, and otherwise immersed in Nepal's deaf society. In Maunabudhuk and Bodhe, along with attending the NSL class each morning, I took part in the everyday rhythms of bazaar life, and, with Sagar, made frequent visits to deaf interlocutors' homes, most located in the farmland surrounding the bazaar. In accordance with local etiquette, I would bring a gift of food items such as biscuits, and our hosts would serve a snack such as sliced cucumbers rubbed with salt and chili peppers accompanied by tea or alcohol. I cooed over children and admired livestock, listened to parents worry about their children's futures, laughed when others made subtle and not-so-subtle jokes about marriage and sex (and made a few myself), and protested that, really, I could not eat another bite or drink another sip. At times, my fieldwork involved filming or even, on rare occasions, formal linguistic elicitation. Most often it looked like hanging out.

Through these years of engagement, I have become fluent in Nepali Sign Language and, to a somewhat lesser degree, spoken Nepali. I also have gained a great deal of experience communicating in natural sign, both in Kathmandu (especially with older people) and even more so in Maunabudhuk and Bodhe. My fieldwork and the processes of learning to communicate across languages and modalities are inextricable from the fact that I am a hearing person, as I explore more below.

ENTANGLEMENTS

My understanding of the central themes of this text—the relationships between language and sociality, the responsibilities people have for and to one another—has been indelibly marked by loving and being loved in particularly deaf/Nepali ways. To put this concretely: I recall going out for Tibetan food one evening in 2009 or 2010 with two deaf Nepali friends, whom I had known since 2002, along with two hearing American friends from the Fulbright program, whom I had met more recently. Throughout the meal, punctuating our lively conversations, the two Nepali men repeatedly advised the two American women on how to consume their soup such that they would neither spill it nor burn themselves. Eventually one of the women said to me in exasperation, "Tell them we've eaten soup before!"

I must not have ordered soup that night, because I was also frequently the recipient of what NSL signers call ADVICE, from both deaf and hearing Nepalis: sometimes about mundane matters such as how to hand-wash clothes (which, having grown up with a washing machine, I very much appreciated—the first few times) but also on more serious matters. In late 2010, for example, my deaf *bhāi* 'younger brother' chastised me for swearing, explaining that it made me seem crass and inappropriate. This made me cry, which made him cry, but he explained that it was meaningless to have made each other siblings if he didn't actually uphold the responsibilities of that relationship. Similarly, I watched deaf people advise each other on when and how to work, what forms of gossip to ignore, how to behave when interacting with people of different genders, and so forth.

These forms of advice are reminiscent of what Trawick (1990) writes about her involvement in a Tamil family's daily affairs. When one of the women with whom Trawick lived advised her not to look at Trawick's own son too lovingly, lest doing so cause harm, Trawick (1990:93) told her that "it was our custom to let people lead their own lives." Trawick writes, "She said simply, '*Tappu* [That is a mistake].' After some time I learned that if you cared about people, you would interfere" (ibid., brackets in original). I too was swept into a world where withholding one's opinion or knowledge is asocial, where people are expected to "interfere" as a form of ethical engagement. I experienced this as both the recipient of sometimes uncomfortable advice and as the advice-giver. When I first arrived in Maunabudhuk, for example, Sagar was spending most of class time teaching the Nepali alphabet in written and signed modalities. I mentioned to him one day that another deaf teacher I knew taught NSL signs first and then the written and fingerspelled versions. Although I did not directly suggest that Sagar change his methods, he began to spend more time on signs, implying that class was more enjoyable that way. At the time, I rationalized my "interference" in my fieldnotes by noting that prior to his first teaching assignment (he had taught NSL courses in rural areas twice before), Sagar was scheduled to go to Kathmandu for teacher training but a *bandh* 'strike, shutdown' had prevented him from doing so. I would now say that the ethical imperatives of deaf society to participate, not only observe, and to share knowledge (Friedner 2015) overrode my concerns about interfering with his teaching, concerns that are themselves grounded in problematic notions of difference and observational neutrality.

Giving advice to others, taking responsibility for their conduct and sociality, is by no means restricted to deaf people nor to Nepalis, as my mention of Trawick's fieldwork with hearing Indians suggests. Nevertheless, deaf people I knew frequently *framed* it as a particularly deaf duty, a point I explore at greater length in chapter 1. As a brief example, once my friend Dawa Gurung and I ate at a Tibetan restaurant in Thamel, a neighborhood in Kathmandu, and she drove me home on her new scooter. As I described in my fieldnotes: "I told her that she could drop me off at the intersection where you turn to the house, but she drove me all the way, and then said, 'It's dark, deaf people help.'"

This anecdote also points to my own sometimes ambiguous status as a hearing participant in deaf society. As I wrote in my fieldnotes at the time: "I'm not sure if she meant that deaf people help their friends, or that deaf people help each other, where I was in the category of *deaf* as in 'people who sign and are close to me.'"[24] She certainly might have been emphasizing that deaf people consider it important to help others, whether deaf or hearing, Nepali or foreigner, and are capable of doing so. At the same time, the category *deaf* can sometimes encompass people who would not be considered deaf as individuals. NSL signers often use the sign DEAF in ways that function very much like a plural pronoun (usually "we," sometimes "they"), to refer to deaf Nepalis or deaf people in general, to a particular group of deaf people, or even to a group of deaf people that might include hearing people (e.g., a deaf sports team and the interpreters who accompany them).

Friedner (2015) and Kusters (2012b) write about how notions of DEAF DEAF SAME or deaf similitude across difference shape their work as deaf anthropologists studying deaf sociality, while Dikyuva et al. (2012) and Hou (2013) emphasize the importance of involving deaf linguists in sign language documentation and analysis. To be clear, neither Friedner nor Kusters claim to be insiders in the communities in which they work. On the contrary, they pay keen attention to questions of national, class, educational, and racial differences, problematizing the notion of DEAF SAME while analyzing its effects. More recently, Friedner (2022) has also explored her complicated position conducting research on cochlear implants (CIs) as a deaf person with a CI who both speaks and signs.

Here, I want to think through the specificity of conducting research as a hearing, signing person in deaf worlds. As a white, Jewish, hearing woman from the United States who signs and speaks, I am very clearly "different" from my interlocutors. Yet I frequently had linguistic relationships with deaf people—particularly NSL signers—that my hearing interlocutors did not have and vice versa. Both speech and sign are understood in deaf society as valuable, and NSL signers with whom I spent time often recognized and appreciated that I was learning, or had learned, NSL. NSL-signing deaf friends not infrequently asked me to interpret in informal situations—with shopkeepers, on a phone call, or even with family members. This relationship was not unilateral, as NSL signers also served as interpreters for me—for example, with NEW signers (deaf people who had recently started to learn NSL) and deaf natural signers—and tended to be deeply patient accommodating my NSL learning process. On occasion, my deaf friends would instruct me not to speak when we were in hearing-majority spaces so they could negotiate the situation as cultural experts. My point is not to reify, nor to simplify, power imbalances or differences but rather to acknowledge that my abilities to speak and sign with deaf and hearing people were often unique in a given setting, a point some of my hearing and deaf friends explicitly made.

In Maunabudhuk these dynamics of ambiguous sameness and difference further intensified because I was the only NSL signer other than Sagar living there at the time. While Sagar and hearing villagers frequently communicated directly (usually in natural sign, and less often in written Nepali), at other times I was asked to translate. He also asked me to monitor whether hearing people said the word *lāṭo*, the Nepali word often used to refer to deaf people that NSL signers consider derogatory. Similarly, while I often communicated directly with deaf natural signers, Sagar often translated for me to help me understand, especially in the earlier months. I would sometimes tell him what a hearing person had said and he would offer further background and context to help me understand more fully.

Translation was in fact a ubiquitous dimension of my fieldwork, and not only across sensory differences. For example, I had an affectionate relationship with the hearing husband of Sanu Kumari Limbu, an older woman who participated in the NSL class in Maunabudhuk. Nevertheless we had difficulty understanding each other, and on one occasion a young Nepali speaker "translated" between us, with all three of us speaking Nepali. Translational practices were not unfamiliar to this multilingual family. According to Sanu Kumari's youngest daughter's husband, a man from the Rai ethnic group, Sanu Kumari's husband would translate between Sanu Kumari and the son-in-law because Sanu Kumari doesn't speak Rai or Nepali and her son-in-law doesn't sign or speak Limbu.[25]

My requests for translations of natural sign had several motivations. Especially in the beginning of my time in Maunabudhuk, I often asked Sagar to translate what local signers were saying to help me to understand in the immediate context and to learn local sign conventions. In addition, I asked hearing people to translate, sometimes because I hadn't understood and also to get a sense of what other people understood—that is, as a methodological tool.[26] I did not want to assume that my own understanding was necessarily representative of others'; one way I sought to calibrate my understanding with that of others was by asking for translation. These requests sometimes provided information that I found useful/instructive: translations, or a clear sense that a hearing interlocutor did or did not understand what a deaf signer was saying. However, as I discuss in chapter 5, instances of requested translation are conversational moves, often producing explicit social assessments of understanding and not-understanding that might not have been uttered in the absence of such a request.

DOING FIELDWORK IN AND WRITING ABOUT NATURAL SIGN

While self-reflexive questions about understanding are frequently foregrounded in anthropological practice, in my fieldwork I was constantly asking not only if I had understood but also if others had, sometimes at the most basic level of reference. This and related questions have followed me through the process of analyzing my fieldnotes and video recordings: *Did he understand her? Is it because she used a sign he couldn't interpret, because natural sign doesn't include a conventional way to say something, or because he looked away in frustration? Given that natural sign is both something learned and something always emergent, how might I know for sure?* Translation is never a simple process, but asking for or giving translations in languages like NSL or Nepali often felt fairly smooth, while asking others to translate natural sign often raised significant additional questions. *Why did she say she could understand and then tell me she couldn't translate what was said? Why did she say she couldn't understand but then respond?*

Watching and conversing with natural signers in Maunabudhuk, Bodhe, Kathmandu, and elsewhere, as well as with NSL signers using natural sign, I frequently have found myself in awe of how people communicate, casually, easily, and effectively, in the absence of what most people in the world think of and experience as language, whether spoken or signed. In months of living in Maunabudhuk, I saw natural sign used among deaf people and between deaf and hearing people to exchange news, make jokes, negotiate work arrangements, discuss national politics, curse, flirt, argue, describe past, ongoing, and hypothetical events, evaluate others' internal states, tell stories, express worries, and wonder about the future. But I have also watched a deaf signer try to communicate something that clearly existed in her mind and that she *knew* she was representing with her signs—and yet her addressees, including me, could not grasp it. I have watched people—more often hearing, but occasionally deaf—act dismissive toward, or get bored trying to understand, a natural signer. I have found myself seduced by the ease of conventional language too, my attention shifting from a more laborious conversation in natural sign to an easier one in NSL in situations where both NSL and natural signers were present. Using natural sign, I have tried to make myself understood, and both succeeded and failed; I have tried to make sense of others, and both succeeded and failed. I felt frustration in the field, shame, anger; I felt joy, admiration, pleasure.

My experiences of learning natural sign through spending time with natural signers, of communicating in it, and of failing to communicate in it—the phenomenology of using natural sign, the corporeality, the surrounding emotions—deeply inform the way I write about it. At the same time, I am wary of falling into the trap of assuming that my experiences, and particularly my failures, actually belong to another, whether a person or a communicative mode. This wariness is informed by the history of a vast array of refusals by scholars and others to recognize the fullness, complexity, or linguistic status of non-Western languages, signed languages, and otherwise marginalized languages. Thus it becomes critical that I observed other people struggle to communicate in natural sign as well. Deaf residents often but not always understood each other. Sagar was able to communicate with hearing villagers in ways many deaf local signers could not and with deaf villagers in ways many hearing local signers could not. But he too came up against dead ends. In many instances, deaf natural signers and their family members could communicate more effectively with each other than I could; in others, it seemed to me that I was able to understand their utterances better than they could each other's. And as mentioned, my requests for translation sometimes ended up drawing my attention to the limits of deaf local signers' hearing interlocutors' own understanding.

These and other tensions were present in the field and they continue to animate my writing. It is vitally important to me not to dismiss or pathologize the brilliant ways the people I work with communicate, as people in similar positions have often been framed as "having no language," as Moriarty (2019) argues; part of how I work to do this is to focus my analysis on situated interactions that inevitably reveal complex, interpersonal sense-making processes. The desire to recognize the facility and inventiveness of deaf signers is also part of what motivates my choice not to use the framework of language deprivation, despite its importance in contemporary research and politics. The concept of language deprivation, or linguistic deprivation, is rooted in the fields of psychology and education, and both highlights and theorizes the many kinds of harm done when deaf people—in particular, but not only, children—do not have access to signing or other accessible language, negatively impacting their communication, their familial, educational, and social experiences, and their physical and mental health (Humphries et al. 2016; Hall 2017; Hall, Levin, and Anderson 2017; Kushalnagar et al. 2020).

In many instances deaf people are actively denied access to signing because of what is known as oralism: ideologies and practices that promote, enact, and institutionalize ideas that speech is superior to sign, that learning to sign precludes learning to speak, and that deaf people should be forbidden to sign (Baynton 1996; Jokinen 2000; Ladd 2003). In other situations schools provide (variably proficient) sign interpreters—but to students who have not had the opportunity to learn a signed language and who continue to be surrounded by nonsigners (Caselli, Hall, and Henner 2020). Work on language deprivation is closely related to work on what is called late language acquisition: when deaf people learn a conventional signed language after childhood (e.g., Mayberry 2010), because they had been kept from it purposefully and/or because it was socially/geographically unavailable.[27]

Deaf and hearing scholars and activists raise these issues to support the critical need for deaf children to have early, consistent access to signers who are fluent in the locally relevant signed language(s) (e.g., Humphries et al. 2013). As several friends and colleagues have impressed upon me, the concept of language deprivation is a powerful tool for fighting *against* ableism, audism, and the suppression and delegitimation of sign, and *for* the flourishing of deaf socialities, signing practices, and sign-centered spaces—efforts with which I fully align.

Language deprivation is not, however, a framework that I encountered locally, although I discuss some parallels with NSL signers' discourse; moreover, I hesitate to call any particular person with whom I worked "language deprived." It is important to me to describe my interlocutors' creative and agentive communicative practices. It is equally important to me not to smooth over the rough patches; not to pretend that I did not see people who were lonely and in pain at least in part because others would or could not understand them—and I seek to give emphasis to the role of addressees and to both the "would not" and "could not." It is my desire to do justice to the complexities of what I experienced, what others allowed me to experience with them, that shapes my writing. The tension between recognizing the ways that signers outside of conventional signed language communities communicate and recognizing the vulnerabilities they face is shaped by long histories inside and outside of academia of both suppressing sign and dismissing communicative practices that look unfamiliar. I am thinking here with scholars such as De Meulder (2019), De Meulder et al. (2019), Henner and Robinson (2023), and Goico and Horton (2023), as well as with friends and colleagues who generously shared their perspectives on this and related tensions.[28] It is certainly possible that some of the experiences I describe in this book might be productively thought of in terms of language deprivation. I have chosen in this book, however, to frame and theorize natural signers' experiences by focusing on semiotic affordances and constraints, and on ethical orientations, acknowledging and analyzing both the possibilities that natural signers create and the precarities they encounter.

This book is not a lament or a celebration, but it both laments and celebrates.

WRITING FOR DIVERSE AUDIENCES, OR WHY THERE IS NO *WE*

The specificity of the communicative practices I write about shapes how I think about my audience. When scholars write about many communicative practices, they can assume that their readers have some familiarity with the general type of subject matter—for example, conversations, debates, love letters, songs—and as Bill Hanks (pers. comm.) argues, in those cases, the challenge is to bring awareness to what usually goes unnoticed. Even when researchers write about conventional signed languages for audiences that include nonsigners, they can rely on those readers' experiences of conventional spoken language and co-speech gesture—not, of course, that signed languages are reducible to either of these, nor to the two in combination. In these cases the figure of analysis takes its shape not only in relation to the ground of analysis but also in relation to the reader's ground of experience. With natural sign, however, for many of my readers the text alone will constitute the ground.

You may have noticed that I avoid the use of the rhetorical *we* in this book. I do so in order to minimize my assumptions about readers' experiences. It is important to me that this book be meaningful—though perhaps differently so—to readers who have never communicated in natural sign or anything resembling it, or perhaps in any signed mode at all, as well as to those who have, and I expect that the experience of reading this will be very different for these two broad groups. Particularly for the former, there may be moments in the book when an earlier point only becomes clear in retrospect. Such moments are inevitable in all language use, and perhaps especially common in natural sign: what comes later clarifies, narrow downs, or amplifies what came before. Imagine this book as a conversation: someone standing at a table points vaguely into the next room, and says, "Can you get one more?" She then glances around at the number of people gathered (five) and the number of chairs (four). Suddenly everything becomes clear: she is pointing at, and asking for, another chair, not the bucket beside it or the sweater on top of it. In those moments just before things come together, I ask patience of the former set of readers. At other times, I will engage in description that may seem interestingly familiar (I hope) or boringly obvious (I hope not) to the latter set of readers, and at those times I ask for their patience.

The fundamentally relational nature of intelligibility in general but more specifically in natural sign also has impacted how I write. By definition, ethnographic engagement is cooperative action (Goodwin 2018). The anthropologist is involved in what she studies (Trawick 1990; Hou 2020), and this truism is heightened when communication is particularly profoundly contingent on the parties involved, as in the case of natural sign. I am quite present in the text, as a reader of a very early version of this book pointed out. My goal isn't to draw attention to myself per se but rather to remind the reader of my presence—as participant, as writer— in order to give a more nuanced and robust account. I am invested in trying to describe and present the messiness, the complicatedness, the irreducible relationality of the phenomena I'm writing about, even when that makes for more tentative claims. I appear quite a lot, and I often appear unsure, hesitant, caught up in the process of sense-making rather than necessarily holding out something definitive that I have already made sense of for you, the reader. This is especially apparent when I offer you the uncertainty contained in my fieldnotes or a series of possible interpretations of something that happened.

GUIDE TO CHAPTERS

Chapter 1 offers an account of how my fieldwork with NSL signers shaped my approach to natural sign. Arguing that NSL signers experience language as radically contingent both collectively and individually, I analyze NSL metalinguistic categories and discourses to show that NSL signers posit NSL and natural sign as similar in some ways but also distinct. I explore NSL signers' critiques of the vernacular Nepali term *lāṭo*, which strongly connotes unintelligibility and is frequently used to refer to deaf people. NSL signers challenge both the word and the logic of hearing people who use it, emphasizing that intelligibility is situational. NSL signers acknowledge that all deaf people experience communicative vulnerability but emphasize that it is far more common for natural signers, on whom the remainder of the book focuses.

Chapter 2 moves to Maunabudhuk, the village that hosted a six-month NSL class in 2010, and the adjacent village of Bodhe. The first half of the chapter queries what *deaf* means in this setting, both to deaf and hearing people, and demonstrates that both *deaf* and *hearing* have socioculturally specific meanings. The second half of the chapter focuses on the demographics of Maunabudhuk and Bodhe. It shows how from the standpoint of social, spatial, and generational relationships among deaf people and between deaf and hearing people, it is unsurprising that natural sign conversations can be both robust and fragile.[29] This chapter also argues that natural sign, as a mode of ever-emergent language, both exceeds the boundaries of familiar scholarly categories of signed communication and demands recognition that at least in some times and places, the world has always been deaf and hearing.

Deepening the analysis of natural sign's paradoxical nature as explored in chapters 1 and 2, chapter 3 both posits and troubles the boundary between linguistic and other sociomaterial conventions. The immanence of natural signs enables a great deal to be said and understood, both with and beyond (or before) linguistic conventions, while the leanness of those conventions and the work required to wrest immanence into actuality mean that that neither signers nor analysts can assume automatic understanding. This chapter revisits the concept of *emergence* to think about how people put together pieces of utterances to make meaning, drawing on grammatical and pragmatic conventions, immediate linguistic and material contexts, and relevant social and cultural knowledge. While both conventional and emergent language users do this, natural sign tips heavily toward less routinized and more labor-intensive modes of sense-making.

Building on these analyses of the demographic and semiotic characteristics of natural sign, chapter 4 argues that interlocutors' orientations are foundational to the interactional production of intelligible utterances and persons. I track willingness and refusal through eye gaze, the production of signs, evaluations of understanding, and spoken Nepali translations, showing how shifting and often contradictory stances reflected and instantiated in these actions (re)produce a world in which understanding natural sign is always in question. Within this world deaf signers must work to try to secure the attention of their hearing interlocutors, who are only sometimes willing to look and to make sense of what they see.

Chapter 5 further explores what *understanding* means, methodologically, socially, and analytically. How did my fieldwork affect the very processes I sought to, well, understand? Are there particular kinds of topics that are especially prone to misunderstandings? How does partial understanding get transformed into misunderstanding or not-understanding or into engaged understanding? This chapter also addresses the long-term sedimentation of precarious communication in individual deaf people's lives and in the figure of the deaf person as *lāṭo*. The afterword reflects on translation, on love, and on why this book matters, and offers an alternative kind of sense-making, describing how deaf people engage with each other even when they have not fully understood what someone else has signed.

PART ONE

Natural Sign and Natural Signers

1

Deaf Theory

This chapter is about signing, but it begins with a request regarding written words. In late spring 2010 in Maunabudhuk, the village in eastern Nepal that was hosting a six-month Nepali Sign Language (NSL) class for deaf adults, staff members at the government health post painted information pertaining to mothers' and children's health on the outside walls of the building. In bright red letters the post warned that maternal vitamin and mineral deficiencies could cause babies to be born deaf or intellectually disabled. The Nepali word that I have represented in the previous sentence with the English word *deaf* is *lāṭo*, which means something like 'dumb' in both the senses of unintelligent and mute (and unfortunately I did not record the Nepali word that I have represented with the English phrase 'intellectually disabled').

Unsurprisingly, when Sagar Karki, the deaf NSL teacher with whom I worked closely, saw what had been written, he was upset. Like many NSL signers, Sagar considers *lāṭo* to be an insulting, inappropriate, and inaccurate way to refer to deaf people. Enlisting me to interpret, Sagar approached the staff and convinced them to paint over *lāṭo* and write *bahirā* instead, a word that more neutrally refers to someone who does not hear. His actions articulated with long-term efforts by deaf and disability leaders to replace derogatory spoken and written Nepali words for disabled people with neutral terminology. For the purposes of this chapter, Sagar's response to the word *lāṭo* offers an entry point into NSL signers' understandings of sociality, language, and communication—understandings that have shaped my own approach to understanding natural sign.[1]

NSL signers' theories arise from their experiences of being signers of a young language and also from their experiences of moving between NSL and natural sign, or between what I refer to as conventional and emergent language. While common for NSL signers, and not radically dissimilar from those of many deaf signers elsewhere in the world, these experiences are unusual when compared with the unmarked subjects of social theory: hearing people who grow up using the language(s) of their communities. Bringing together the commitments of deaf studies and anthropology to recognizing the enormous debts that academic knowledge production owes to the intellectual labor of people with whom academics work, I think of NSL signers' insights as a kind of uncommon commonsense that deserves documentation and explication both in its own right and in relation to the theory-building it has helped me to produce.

The chapter begins with a section that briefly sketches the historical emergence of NSL and deaf society to provide context for NSL signers' (un)commonsense understandings of language and sociality. For NSL signers, both NSL itself and the ease of understanding and being understood that NSL makes possible are contingent historically, biographically, and in everyday life. These contingencies produce an experiential tension: NSL both is and is not necessary for deaf signers to engage in communicative sociality. This tension appears in the language's referential structure and in NSL signers' characterizations of natural sign. Exploring these terms and characterizations leads to analyzing deaf NSL signers' sense of their responsibilities toward other deaf people. I show that NSL signers identify how hearing people exclude deaf signers from communicative sociality not only because hearing people do not know NSL but also because they do not bother to use or understand natural sign. This lack of motivation and action both produces and is produced by the figure of deaf people as *lāṭo* to which Sagar objected. Finally, I describe ways of talking about deaf people in speech and sign; examine NSL signers' critiques of the word *lāṭo* and the attitudes and actions of people who use it; and analyze ambiguities in those critiques that point to the ethical and social labor that conventional language does for its users.

A BRIEF HISTORY OF THE PRESENT

Community narratives ground NSL signers' collective history—the history of the emergence of NSL and deaf society—in the founding of Nepal's first permanent school for the deaf in 1966 (Sharma 2003; Green 2014c; Hoffmann-Dilloway 2016). In NSL the school is referred to with the sign NAXAL, the Kathmandu neighborhood where it is currently located, and I refer to it henceforth as Naxal or the Naxal school. From 1966 until 1988 the school adhered to a strict oralist philosophy (Joshi 1991; Prasad 2003): the use of sign was banned and students were required to learn speech and lip-reading. Acharya (1997:1, quoted in Hoffmann-Dilloway 2016:47), a former Naxal student, remembers that if students signed, "the teachers would scold us, hold our hands down, twist our ears, and pull our hair." Neither the policy nor the teachers' actions, however, stopped the young deaf students from signing.

Years later, these signers would still recall meeting up for the pleasure of using their hands to talk. As Acharya (1997:4, quoted in Hoffmann-Dilloway 2016) describes: "When 1:00 came, the time for tiffin, the students could surreptitiously communicate through visual and gestural modalities. After 4:00 in the afternoon we were free to talk to each other using signs after leaving school. There was no particular reason to return home early if we did not have to, since we were not able to communicate effectively with our families. So we would gather in a specific place after school to socialize using sign language until 7 or 8 in the evening." Another former student, slightly younger than Acharya, described the making of NSL to me in similar terms, mentioning the importance of both school and the Kathmandu Association of the Deaf (KAD), founded in 1980 by a group of former Naxal students and usually considered the first deaf-run association in the country.[2] I wrote in my fieldnotes: "There was the younger crowd of school boys, who weren't allowed to sign and had to sign only on the sly—they'd set times and places after school and they would meet to let their hands go crazy, signing and signing. There was also the older crowd who founded the Kathmandu Association of the Deaf. As [my friend] told it, these two groups eventually merged, and with this merging came the formation of NSL."[3]

According to deaf narratives, NSL grew out of the communicative interactions of several cohorts of deaf children and young adults who spent their days together at the Naxal school and later at KAD. Presumably, in the earlier years especially, they began by communicating in what today NSL signers call NATURAL-SIGN (Green 2014c). There is also evidence that one or more Nepali students had spent time in India learning Indian Sign Language (Hoffmann-Dilloway 2016:47, citing Sharma 2003, and Arjun Shrestha, pers. comm.). Deaf schools often figure as the birthplace of a language and deaf community. As Padden (2011) argues, signing practices often already exist in the places where deaf schools are established *and* deaf schools bring together the critical mass of signers theorized as necessary for the emergence of signed languages. Friedner (2015) has theorized that deaf educational spaces give rise to and are cultivated as moral spaces where deaf people orient, and are encouraged to orient, toward each other. Bringing together Padden's and Friedner's work with the emphasis on attention and responsibility that NSL signers articulate, it becomes clear that deaf schools produce language not only because of the number of deaf people present but also because of their desire and willingness to make sense to and of each other.

In 1995 leaders from KAD and seven other regional deaf organizations formed what is now known as the National Federation of the Deaf Nepal (abbreviated NDFN). Over the years the number of local deaf associations has steadily grown. In late 2010, NDFN had twenty-five member chapters; at the time of writing, the organization's website states that there are fifty-three.[4] The growth of deaf-run institutions over the past few decades has both produced and been produced by growing numbers of educational facilities for the deaf. As of 2011, at least 18 deaf schools and more than 125 deaf classes (within hearing schools) were operating in nearly all of Nepal's then-75 districts (Hundley 2011). The NSL term DEAF SCHOOL includes both schools and classes, and many deaf classes, like deaf schools, offer residential facilities and serve a similar—though differently scaled—function, bringing deaf children into the wider network of deaf NSL signers.[5]

At a program in 2006, NDFN's president at the time, Bikash Dangol, emphasized the importance of deaf schools. Addressing an audience of deaf activists, parents of deaf children, and hearing functionaries, he argued that establishing schools for the deaf is more urgent than establishing schools for the hearing, because hearing children who don't attend school still have a social education. From the perspective of deaf NSL signers, going to school is not only about acquiring skills such as Nepali, and increasingly English, literacy but also, and more fundamentally, about acquiring a conventional language and being part of deaf society. Deaf society includes and extends beyond schools; it is the always-growing network of (primarily) NSL signers who come together at formal and informal events, within and across particular places.[6]

During my fieldwork in Kathmandu, deaf people could be found every day of the week but Saturday at KAD. People would drop by not only for official business but also to spend time with their friends or catch up on news; organizations elsewhere, such as the Gandaki Association of the Deaf in Pokhara, serve a similar function. The ever-expanding Bakery Café chain offers another kind of "deaf space" (Gulliver 2006, cited in Kusters 2015), as it hires many deaf waiters, providing a steady paycheck for work done in the company of other signers, as well as facilitating interactions between deaf and hearing people (Hoffmann-Dilloway 2011b). District-level associations as well as the NDFN hold yearly meetings and cultural events such as dance performances and picnics, facilitate vocational training programs, and work with foreign NGOs, while deaf sports organizations coordinate games within the country and abroad. Outside of schools and other institutions, friends get together at homes and tea shops, in soccer fields and restaurants. They invite each other to celebrate birthdays, rice feedings, and weddings. Indeed, marriages between deaf sweethearts are now common. Deaf Nepalis have forged both durable spaces and iterative events in which they come together, on local, regional, national, and international levels. However, NSL signers do not claim that communicative sociality is *only* available in NSL.

THREE LEVELS OF CONTINGENCY

Whereas users of Nepali, or for that matter natural sign, cannot point to a specific person and say, "That person helped make our language," among NSL signers, doing this is not just possible but common. This is the first level on which NSL signers experience the contingency of NSL and deaf society. The oldest users of NSL—sometimes called the first cohorts or generations in scholarship on young signed languages—are alive and known by other NSL signers, often through their positions as leaders in deaf organizations. Individuals' biographies constitute the second level of contingency. Unlike hearing people who learn spoken language from birth, many, perhaps most, deaf NSL signers can remember learning NSL. They often can point, rhetorically and literally, to people from whom they learned NSL, people whom they helped learn NSL, and/or people who helped them or whom they helped to access the spaces where they learned it.[7] For example, a decade after learning NSL at the age of sixteen, my friend Sommaya Lama continued to refer to the woman who had first taught her in precisely those terms. Relatedly, in NSL spaces people frequently asked me, "Who taught you NSL?" (In the United States, I am more likely to be asked *why* or *how* I learned ASL.) Even if the person questioning me did not immediately recognize the name of my first NSL teacher, the form of my response—my teacher's name, which I would usually offer first as a name sign and then sometimes fingerspell with the NSL alphabet— served to place me in a constellation of personal connections.

In an inverse of both the first and second levels, most if not all NSL signers personally know deaf adults who either do not know NSL at all or are learning it in the present: perhaps a deaf neighbor or older relative, whether someone from Kathmandu or someone who traveled there from a more rural area, where there are fewer deaf schools and organizations. As I argue in Green 2014c (35–39), NSL signers' characterizations of cities and villages reflect broader (hearing) tropes about development and space (Pigg 1996, 1992; Liechty 2003, 2001) but also reflect irreducibly deaf experiences of language- and locality-specific modes of sociality. It is unmistakable for NSL signers that things could have been different. Alternative histories are close by, embodied in persons.

In a 2012 interview, Prajwal Dangol, then in his mid-twenties, recalled how excited and disoriented he felt during his first day at Naxal, at the age of eight. He had previously attended an educational program for children with disabilities, but this was his first experience in a signing environment. During the interview Prajwal was sitting next to his former schoolmate, Furba Sherpa, who, Prajwal explained, had started school a year earlier and was repeating the same grade. He continued: "So I was new, and Furba was already a good signer, in fact he was the cleverest kid in class. And I didn't know sign. You know the posters with the NSL alphabet, those were up on the walls, and I just stood staring at them open-mouthed. Furba got my attention and showed me the signs for the letters. I kept looking, and tried to make those signs. I didn't know sign at all. I tried and tried and tried, and I did learn."[8] Prajwal relayed this story with his usual panache, depicting himself staring up at the posters with rapt attention. On the one hand, he told the story as if it were interesting but not remarkable, and indeed, learning conventional language at age eight is not especially unusual among deaf NSL signers. On the other hand, to return to a point made in the introduction, the principal assumptions around sociality and language made by the (hearing) social sciences—with the exception of deaf studies and allied fields—fail to account for such experiences.

In a different context Prajwal reflected further on the importance of (learning) NSL. Discussing with a friend why potential sweethearts should talk directly with each other, Prajwal asked the following question: "You're deaf, I'm deaf, other people are deaf. Do we COMMUNICATE or miscommunicate [literally, MISS]?" Prajwal's friend, also a young man then in his twenties, replied, "We communicate," or more literally, "[Our communication] ALIGNS." In response, Prajwal confirms, "Right, because of *SĀNKETIK BHĀSĀ* 'SIGN LANGUAGE.'" His deployment of a question with an expected answer is a familiar and effective NSL rhetorical device. Its power relies on the response being predictable and uncontested: here, that deaf people communicate. Of course, deaf NSL signers sometimes do miscommunicate with each other, but this is beside the point, because it is *only* with other NSL signers that communication can ever be taken for granted.[9]

Prajwal's claim leads to the third level of contingency. NSL signers' communication aligns with other NSL signers', not with everyone's. In their everyday lives, however, deaf NSL signers must communicate with variously positioned deaf and hearing people; Graif (2018) also addresses this theme. My friend Sommaya, for example, used NSL with other NSL signers, and mixtures of speech, mouthing, lipreading, and natural sign when we spent time visiting her parents in Nuwakot and with her sister with whom she lived in Kathmandu. I watched Prajwal charm hearing shopkeepers in natural sign and discuss family issues with his hearing mother in a mixture of NSL, natural sign, and mouthed Nepali and Newari words. In Maunabudhuk, Sagar shifted between signing NSL with me, using natural sign with both hearing and deaf people, writing Nepali with some of his hearing age-mates, and asking me to translate between NSL and spoken Nepali. While NSL signers communicate with people beyond deaf society, sometimes it MISSES and sometimes it ALIGNS.

Next, I discuss how NSL signers refer to and evaluate their own and others' communicative practices and their efficacy, in various ways, depending on the contexts of both communication and evaluation. What I want to emphasize here is that these evaluations are grounded in lifelong, everyday experiences of moving between ways of communicating, calibrating (Moriarty and Kusters 2021) their communication to the specific needs of the situation and their interlocutors (Hiddinga and Crasborn 2011). NSL signers' communicative practices in and across NSL, natural sign, and resources from spoken and written languages mean that deaf NSL signers experience and are keenly aware of an existential tension: conventions matter and communication outside of conventions is possible.

METASIGNS AND METALINGUISTIC DISCOURSE

This tension is reflected in the referential structure of key NSL metasigns (signs about signing) and in metalinguistic discourse about signing. Briefly put, the sign SIGN can refer to signing in general, including NSL and natural sign, and also more narrowly to NSL. Moreover, discursive characterizations of natural sign also convey a kind of ambivalence or multiplicity. NSL signers describe natural

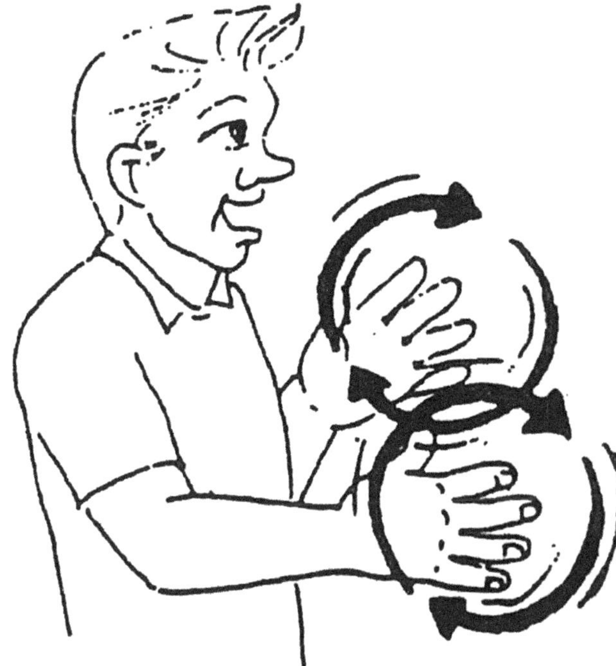

FIGURE 2. The sign SIGN. A person's two open hands face each other and move toward and away from the chest in alternating circles. Illustration by Pratigya Shakya (NDFN 2003:17). Reproduced by permission from the National Federation of the Deaf Nepal (NDFN).

sign as restricted and restricting yet expansive, as "smaller than NSL" but also equivalent to it; as something (at least partly) learned from hearing people and as something that hearing people frequently can't be bothered to partake in.

Key Signs

SIGN comprises an overarching category. Figure 2 shows an illustration by Pratigya Shakya of the sign SIGN; it appears in the NSL dictionary published and distributed by the NDFN that was nearly ubiquitous in NSL signers' homes during my fieldwork (NDFN 2003). SIGN encompasses NSL and natural sign and is also used when talking about foreign sign languages. In contrast, the signed phrase NEPALI SIGN LANGUAGE, as well as shorter versions like NEPALI SIGN or SIGN LANGUAGE, almost always refer specifically to what in this text I call NSL (as with Prajwal's quote earlier). And, as I discuss below, NSL signers refer to NSL most frequently with the sign SIGN.

The sign NATURAL-SIGN refers to communicative practices used by various types of people in various situations, including:

- deaf NSL signers when they communicate with deaf Nepalis who do not know NSL, with hearing Nepalis who do not know NSL, or with deaf or hearing foreigners who do not know NSL;

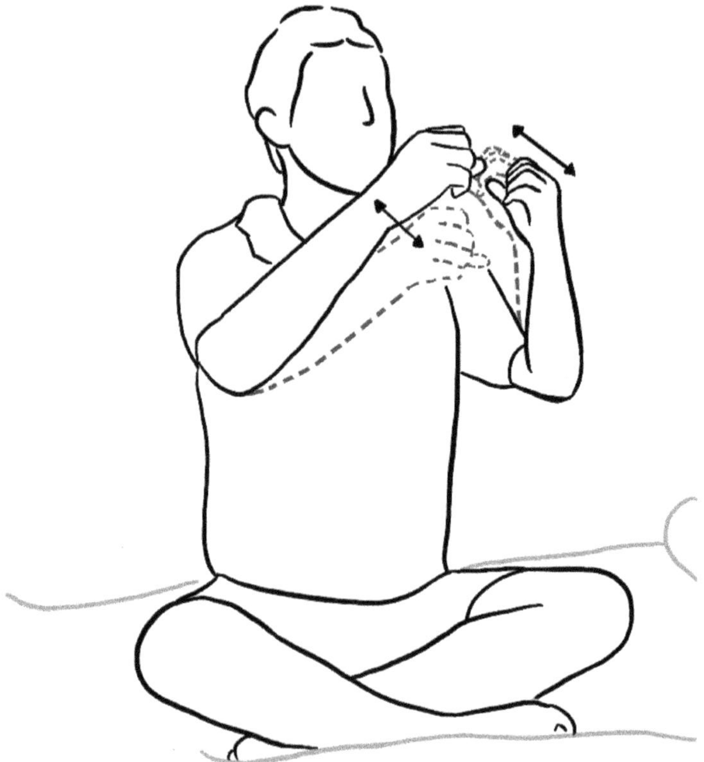

FIGURE 3. Furba Sherpa signs "NATURAL-SIGN": the fingers of each hand touch the inside middle of each thumb; the hands move alternately toward and away from the chest, thumbs brushing as the hands pass each other. Illustration by Nanyi Jiang.

- deaf Nepalis who do not know NSL sign when they communicate with anyone, deaf or hearing;
- hearing Nepalis who do not know NSL when they communicate with deaf Nepalis, whether or not the deaf Nepalis know NSL; and
- hearing NSL signers when they communicate with deaf Nepalis who are not NSL signers.

Natural sign, then, refers to communication that occurs in the signed modality and that is not NSL or a foreign signed language. Figure 3 shows the sign NATURAL-SIGN, illustrated by Nanyi Jiang.[10]

The sign NATURAL-SIGN is an initialized sign; the handshape corresponds to the fingerspelled consonant with which the Nepali word *prakriti* 'nature' begins.

In different contexts the same sign could also be glossed NATURE, as in things like waterfalls and thunderstorms, or ON-ONES-OWN, as when talking about how someone learned a handicraft without instruction or the fact that someone had twins without using assistive reproductive technologies (this latter example is drawn from actual conversation and not meant as a judgment on what counts as "natural" in the realm of reproduction). This second meaning, which emphasizes that something was done (perhaps metaphorically) with one's own hands, without formal instruction or intervention, resonates with how NSL signers characterize natural sign. In an interview I conducted with Sagar Karki, he defined natural sign like this: "NATURAL-SIGN is their own LANGUAGE that they've used their entire lives. Did they grow up going to school? They've never been in their lives. I'm teaching them now, but before, from the time their mothers gave birth to them, they would talk about things, using signs to say that the father had gone somewhere, gone outside. Their communication works. Krishna [a deaf man] and the other deaf people [in Maunabudhuk] grew up understanding this kind of sign. There were no [deaf] schools here then, people didn't know about them."[11]

This emphasis on natural sign as a mode deaf people use to communicate without formal instruction is especially relevant when placed in the context of NSL. While deaf NSL signers no doubt acquire NSL primarily through socialization with other NSL signers, every NSL signer I have ever met has also received formal instruction in NSL (or at least its vocabulary, as noted by Hoffmann-Dilloway 2008), whether at school or a deaf organization—the same places where less formal socialization occurs. In other words, regardless of the actual acquisition process, the socially remarked-on fact is that NSL is learned in the context of formal education, as in Prajwal's description of the first time he encountered NSL. In the same interview he recalled having playful conversations in natural sign with his father and with elderly neighbors. Natural sign, then, is learned (and used) in homes and neighborhoods, in contrast to NSL.[12]

Categories and Characterizations

The existence of the signed phrase NEPALI SIGN LANGUAGE and the sign NATURAL-SIGN makes clear that NSL signers distinguish between these modes of signing. Yet two factors produce a blurring of categories. First, what counts as an example of a given category is subject to social evaluation, as Hoffmann-Dilloway (2011a) shows with regards to natural signers learning NSL. Second, a single sign can refer to more than one category and several different signs can refer to the same category. In everyday conversation the phrase NEPALI SIGN LANGUAGE is not commonly employed; the sign SIGN usually refers to NSL and NSL is usually referred to with the sign SIGN. Yet a person who communicates in natural sign also might be described simply as using SIGN. For example, an NSL signer might answer affirmatively when asked if their parents SIGN, and then do so again when asked if they mean their parents use NATURAL-SIGN. Similarly, Sagar used the sign SIGN almost exclusively when discussing signing that, when asked directly, he considered to be natural sign. The referent of SIGN may be identifiable through context or may remain ambiguous.

It is not only the one-to-many and many-to-one relationships between meta-signs and their referents that contribute to a sense of ambiguity about what exactly natural sign is or what functions it can(not) serve. NSL signers also implicitly and explicitly characterize natural sign both as perfectly adequate for commu-nication—and with a broader range of people than NSL—*and* as imposing lim-its on communication. This framing of natural sign is similar to how Indian Sign Language users in Mumbai describe their use of "gesture" to communicate with hearing people (Kusters dir. 2015; Kusters and Sahasrabudhe 2018). NSL signers portray natural sign as having stable lexical, syntactic, and pragmatic properties and establish rhetorical equivalences between NSL and natural sign and between NSL signers and natural signers. At the same time, NSL signers distinguish between the communicative affordances of NSL and natural sign, and differentiate themselves from natural signers. Natural sign thus emerges as a mode of communication that is simultaneously, and contradictorily, powerful and limited/limiting.

In the aforementioned interview with Prajwal Dangol and Furba Sherpa, Furba compared lexical items used "here" by NSL signers in Kathmandu and "there" by natural signers in the Solu Khumbu region where he was born, calling the latter items both "their own" and "our own." At one point I reminded him of an earlier, unrecorded conversation we had had about the sign SCHOOL as convention-ally signed in Maunabudhuk and in his own village. Furba replied, "Yes. Here, [it is signed] SCHOOL; there [in Maunabudhuk, it is signed], SCHOOL; [and in Solu Khumbu, it is signed] SCHOOL."[13] By reproducing the distinct lexical items used in Kathmandu and two other places, Furba accomplishes two things. By *not* men-tioning that the sign that he produces for "here" is an NSL sign, he demonstrates the degree to which NSL is associated with particular places, such as Kathmandu. At the same time, this lack of mention, and the naming of different signs, sets up a metapragmatic correspondence between NSL and natural sign: that is to say, he represents both NSL and natural sign as communicative practices with stable, repeatable lexical items.

Similarly, several deaf teachers I spent time with explained how they would teach NSL to deaf people through the use of their students' own natural signs. Sagar, for example, reported a conversation between himself and Krishna Gajmer, a deaf resident of Maunabudhuk. Each line includes a fairly literal gloss, followed by a more elaborated translation, with line breaks for ease of reading. The let-ter Q represents the general wh-question sign in natural sign (discussed more in chapter 3); the word "Point" is followed immediately by the person, place, or direction pointed to.

1   KRISHNA, HOUSE Q?
     I asked Krishna, "Where do you live?"
2   Point-downhill.
     He answered, "Downhill."
3   Point-Krishna Q? SACRED-THREAD?
     "And are you Bahun/Chhetri?"
4   BLACKSMITH.
     "No, I'm Kami."[14]

While in these reported utterances, each lexical sign Sagar produces is *also* an NSL sign, our preceding turns have framed the reported conversation as natural sign, a characterization that is reinforced by the formal and pragmatic features of Sagar's second question to Krishna about caste/ethnicity.[15] In NSL the conventional way of asking someone their *jāt* 'caste/ethnicity' is to sign, "*JĀT* WHAT? 'What's your caste/ethnic group?'" In natural sign, at least in Maunabudhuk, the conventional way to ask about someone's caste/ethnicity is to ask if someone is a particular *jāt*. This is done using a conventional naming strategy that draws on typified caste/ethnic practices such as blacksmithing, sewing, (not) drinking alcohol, (not) eating pork, or, as in this example, wearing a sacred thread (Green 2022b). In other words, in NSL a signer directly names the general category (*JĀT*) and requests that the addressee identify their particular caste/ethnic group. In natural sign a signer provides an example of the general category and requests that the addressee provide a confirmation or a correction.

Together, Furba and Sagar demonstrate that natural sign exhibits grammatical and pragmatic conventions, at least some of which vary by location. In doing so, they make an implicit claim that, like knowing/using NSL, knowing/using natural sign involves knowledge or skill. I have also seen NSL signers explain how they use natural sign to teach NSL or proudly describe giving tours to signers from other countries (remember that the category NATURAL-SIGN includes some forms of signing between signers who use different but conventional signed languages). Furthermore, I have seen and been told how NSL signers talk with their family members and neighbors using natural sign. For NSL signers, then, natural sign is powerful; in some senses it is more powerful than NSL in that it enables communication with a wide variety of people.

Relatedly, when I asked Furba if natural sign suffices for complete communication for a deaf person in his village who does not know NSL, he said yes. Yet in the same conversation, when I asked about the difference between NATURAL-SIGN and SIGN (interpreted by Furba to mean NSL, which is indeed how I meant it), he answered like this: "Previously, I didn't know that there are different kinds of sign. Natural sign arises, it's their [Solu Khumbu's] own, and I learned it myself according to what I saw. Later, when I was brought to Kathmandu, I came to understand that signing here is different, Kathmandu has its own signing. It's like the aim of

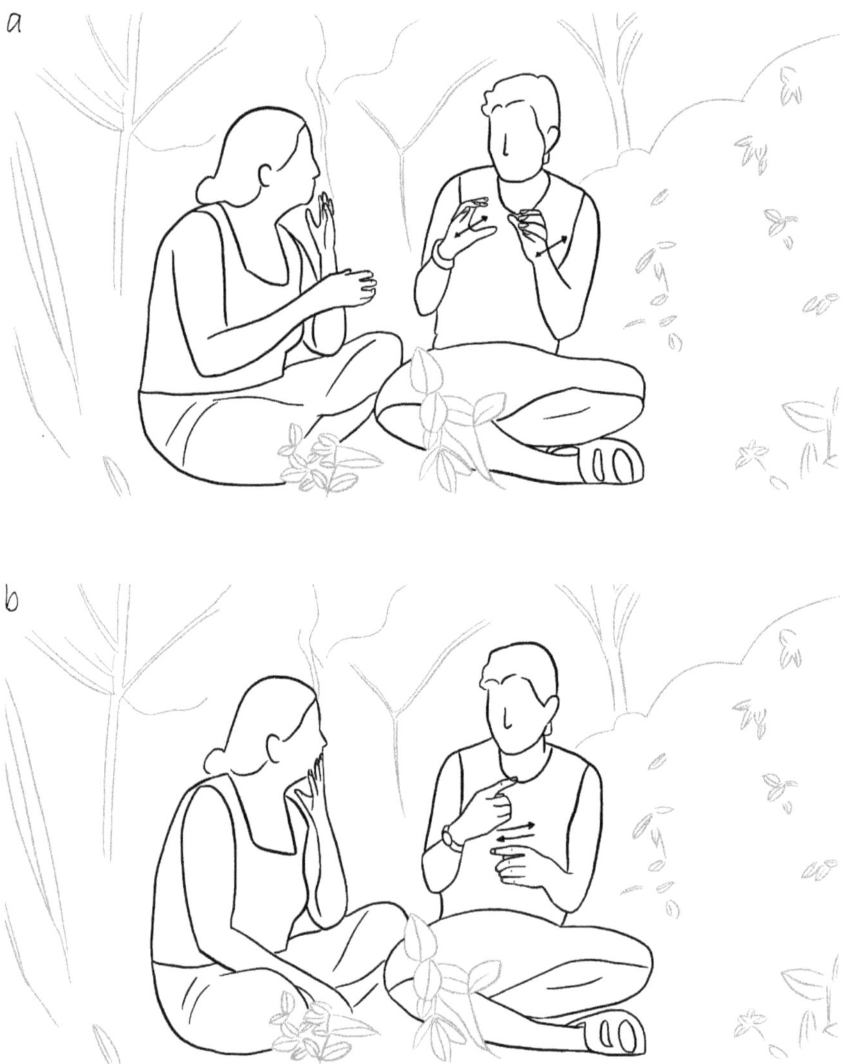

FIGURE 4. (a) Seated in a field next to Mara, Sagar signs "COMMUNICATION," moving two open, curved "C" hands toward and away from his body in alternation. (b) Sagar signs "MISS," moving extended index fingers toward and then past each other. Illustrations by Nanyi Jiang.

NSL is total and complete communication. Natural sign isn't enough. It's smaller."[16] Furba states that as a young deaf child, he acquired natural sign by watching other people. It is ambiguous as to whether the people he was watching were deaf or hearing, but within the discursive logics of NSL signers, it is unlikely that the presence of deaf signers would go unstated. Thus Furba implies that hearing people can use their hands to communicate with someone deaf (and that this is one way deaf children learn natural sign). Such an implication accords with the many times I saw strangers on buses or in stores shift from speaking to signing, or from speaking to speaking and signing, as soon as they realized that their addressee was deaf—and of course does not erase the many ways and times that family members, neighbors, and strangers refused to make adjustments, as explored at length in later chapters. Furba's comments also accord with how Sagar characterizes natural sign as that which deaf people use in conversation with their mothers.

Despite Furba's initial assurance that natural sign is enough, when I ask him to articulate how natural sign is different from NSL, as opposed to taking natural sign on its own terms, he states that natural sign is not sufficient after all, at least not for all communicative purposes. Somewhat inversely, when I asked Sagar if the deaf people with whom he worked could communicate when he first came to Maunabudhuk, at first he said no. Our ensuing conversation makes use of the same contrast between COMMUNICATION MISS (figure 4) and COMMUNI-CATION ALIGN (figure 5) discussed earlier.

Our conversation also demonstrates the ambiguous way that NSL signers talk about natural sign. The numbered lines indicate our alternating turns.

1	Sagar:	No, in the beginning, there was missed communication [COMMU-NICATION MISS].
2	Mara:	So like—
3	Sagar:	When I came here, if I asked where they lived, they would point, or if I asked about their mother or father [using natural signs], they would understand. I have been teaching them, so they have changed [how they sign].
4	Mara:	SIGN and NATURAL-SIGN are different, so there's missed communication, but if you yourself change and put aside sign—
5	Sagar:	I teach using NATURAL-SIGN.
6	Mara:	and use natural sign—from the beginning using natural sign did communication work [COMMUNICATION ALIGN]?
7	Sagar:	Yes
8	Mara:	From the beginning?
9	Sagar:	Yes, it was good. [Like I said] if I asked where they live, they would point. I asked Krishna and he pointed downhill, and I asked if he was Brahman/Chhetri, and he said no, he was Kami. Yeah.
10	Mara:	So from the beginning communication did line up?
11	Sagar:	Only in NATURAL-SIGN.[17]

This translated transcript shows that I had some difficulty specifying what exactly I was asking, no doubt in part because NSL is not my primary language; but I think that Sagar's equivocation also relates to the strong association of the sign COM-MUNICATE with the category of NSL. In NSL discourse good communication is

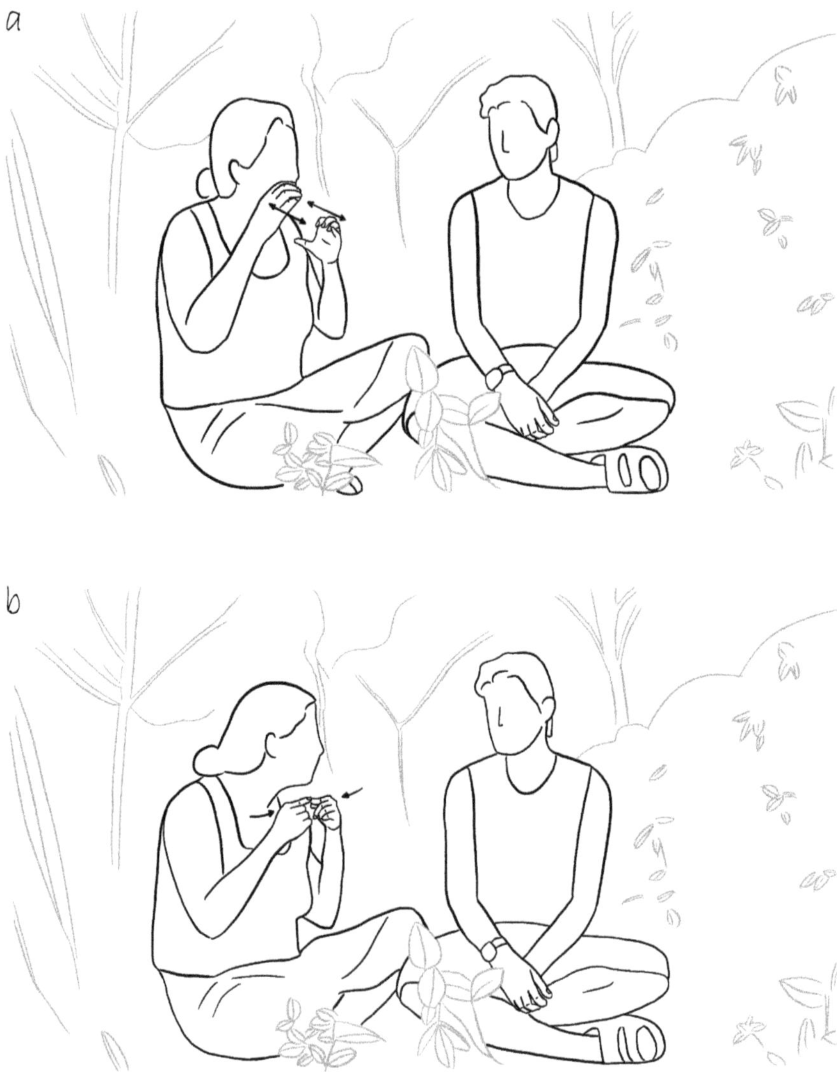

FIGURE 5. (a) Seated in a field next to Sagar, Mara signs "COMMUNICATION," moving two open, curved "C" hands toward and away from her body in alternation. (b) Mara signs "ALIGN," moving extended index fingers toward each other to touch. Illustrations by Nanyi Jiang.

generally understood as what happens in NSL, unless otherwise specified. Yet Sagar positions himself as skilled at code-switching between NSL and natural sign, a facility that I have argued implies some degree of equivalence between the two. This conversation acknowledges that "aligned" communication can happen in natural sign, while also implicitly suggesting the importance of NSL in deaf people's lives.

Deaf NSL signers recognize natural sign as an important and productive communicative mode. At the same time, they frame NSL as central to deaf society—and to the moral imperatives that (should) guide how NSL signers interact with other deaf people. I recall that many years ago a young deaf man told me that he would like to marry a deaf woman "from the hills" to whom he would teach NSL. Institutionally, the imperative to share NSL is operationalized in NDFN-facilitated NSL outreach classes that have been running for decades throughout Nepal, NSL classes offered by district-level deaf organizations, and specialized programs like the Sewing Training Institute for the Deaf for young women as well as the Old Deaf Project for elderly deaf people (Green 2017; Hoffmann-Dilloway 2021), both based in the Kathmandu Valley.

According to Sagar, the NDFN facilitates outreach classes year after year in order to "raise up deaf communication" and ensure equality with hearing people.[18] The intended beneficiaries are not only the students, but also existing members of deaf society. As he said at the concluding program of the Maunabudhuk class, its purpose was also to increase membership in Dhankuta's deaf association.[19] An increase in membership would mean more people to spend time with, more people invested in communicating with each other and in forging connections with other deaf people in Nepal (and beyond). Thus teaching is not only about sharing NSL and deaf-centered values but also about broadening the reach of deaf society.

In this sense, DEAF SOCIETY is both an actually existing network of people and an aspirational project. Deepak Shakya, a founding member of the NDFN and president of the Kathmandu Association of the Deaf at the time, illustrated this duality in his speech at the NDFN's General Assembly program in 2009.[20] Early in his speech he stated that deaf people as signers are equal to hearing people as speakers, then said that deaf people have their own society of which they are all members. He did not specify whether "all" designated every deaf person present or all deaf people in Nepal. Later, he mentioned that although there are many elderly deaf people in Nepal, they were not in attendance at the assembly. He encouraged everyone present not to shun older deaf people, saying that it was important for all deaf people to participate in deaf programs and be part of deaf society. Again, it was not entirely clear whether the point was that old deaf people are part of deaf society or should be. This ambiguity is socially and rhetorically productive, in that it laminates the real and the imperative onto each other.

RESPONSIBILITIES

When discussing both outreach programs and informal interventions, NSL signers not only reiterate the responsibilities that deaf people (should) have for each other; they also imply that deaf people are best suited to teach other deaf people—and not just how to sign NSL, but how to be a person more broadly. During the conversation quoted earlier between Prajwal and his friend, Prajwal turned

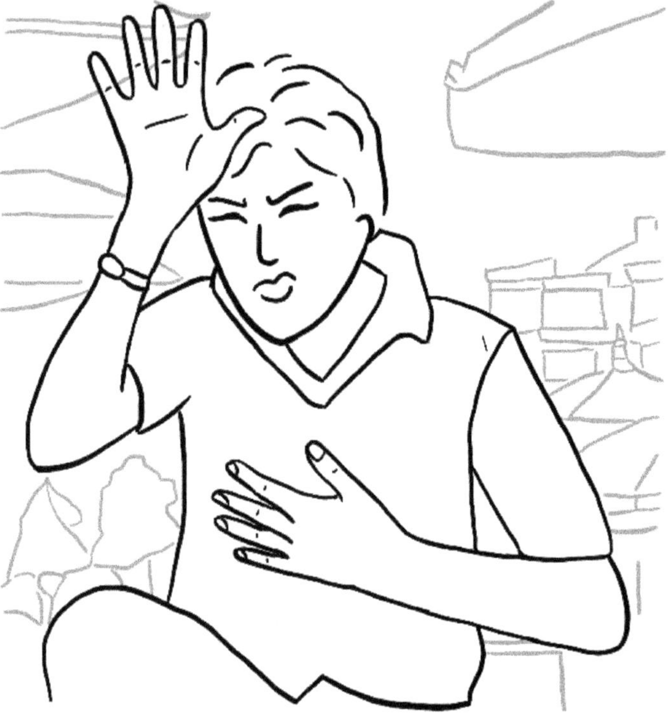

FIGURE 6. Sitting in a plaza, Prajwal demonstrates someone waving their hands meaninglessly; his facial expression is somewhat frustrated. Illustration by Nanyi Jiang.

to the topic of deaf-deaf relationships. He expressed what he would like to say to several deaf acquaintances who he felt were not acting in accordance with norms of deaf unity: "If there's a deaf person flinging their hands around meaninglessly [acting unsocialized or inappropriately; figure 6], you shouldn't push them aside. You should be thoughtful with that person—interrupt them, sit them down, and explain things to them."

At this point Prajwal indicated the friend seated next to him, using him as a real example in the hypothetical conversation playing out. Part way through this next utterance, the imagined addressee shifts from deaf people who are not taking proper care of other deaf people to deaf people who are in need of care. "Just like him, when he was small, he acted the same way, flinging his hands around. I told him not to be like that, I advised him over and over, and he became capable, self-sufficient [literally, he stood up; figure 7]. All of you can too. It won't happen right away, but over time—four years, five years—and with effort, you can.

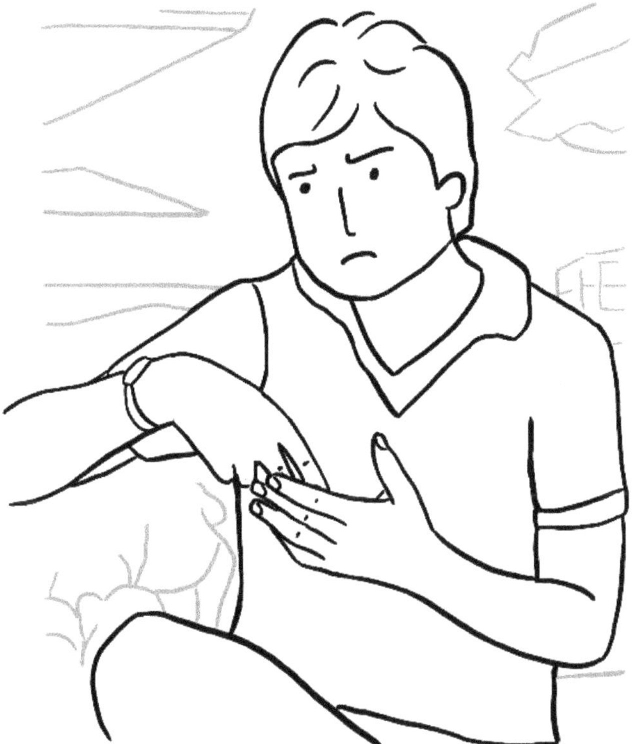

FIGURE 7. Sitting in a plaza, Prajwal signs "TO-BECOME-CAPABLE," planting two fingers of one hand like legs onto his other palm and raising them to stand; his face looks determined. Illustration by Nanyi Jiang.

With him, it was the same. It wasn't just one or two years, but eventually his mind became supple. In the same way, if you try, you all can too."[21]

Prajwal's impromptu lecture clearly articulates how deaf people should act in relation to one another. It also makes explicit a shared understanding that deaf people who are "flinging their hands around meaninglessly" are capable of learning and changing, so long as someone provides the necessary guidance. Moreover, Prajwal was not invoking his friend purely hypothetically. Several months earlier, Prajwal and I were sitting in his house, looking through photographs. One picture featured four young boys: Prajwal, two relatives, and a fourth child, whose appearance—his posture and facial expressions—I associated, rightly or wrongly, with intellectual disability. I asked who he was, and Prajwal replied that he was the deaf friend with whom we had been hanging out earlier. I looked disbelieving, and said that the photo did not resemble him at all, but did not say that he looked intellectually disabled. To my surprise, Prajwal replied, "He looks intellectually disabled, right? He used to be 'half-minded,' and didn't know how to eat or behave and I gave him lots of advice and he turned out fine, and his family was happy."[22] It was this same friend with whom Prajwal was sitting many years later, whom he offered as an example of possible change.

I have struggled with how to think and write about this conversation, because from one perspective it construes intellectual disability as something that should be cured. I take seriously deaf, disabled, and neurodivergent people's resistance against the idea that they need to be fixed, and how a "cure mentality . . . can be a slippery slope toward eugenics when it is applied by abled people" (Moore 2020:76). Yet disability scholars also recognize the tensions and ambivalences of cure (Moore 2020; Clare 2017).[23] And Erevelles (2011, cited in Braswell 2012), Soldatic and Grech (2014), and Nguyen (2018), among others, push back against the way that disability studies frameworks can risk "positioning . . . impairment as natural" (Soldatic and Grech 2014) when in fact some impairment is produced by historical and ongoing systemic inequalities.[24]

Thus I want to take seriously what I understand here as a cautionary tale against "misrecognition," a social phenomenon that Graif (2018:9, 40) argues affects "deaf people worldwide" and very potently in Nepal. While some forms of misrecognition may create more momentary effects, in this case, misrecognition was pervasively limiting the ways that Prajwal's friend could be in the world, because, Prajwal implies, people assumed that his friend was not capable of learning and growing in ways that he in fact was. Presumably if Prajwal or another deaf person had not intervened, the friend would have continued to be treated as he had up to that time. As I understand it, the argument that Prajwal makes here is not that deaf people might not also be intellectually disabled, nor that intellectually disabled deaf people should not also be brought into deaf sociality; rather, it is that different forms of difference should not be conflated, because doing so can harm people. Misrecognition, in other words, has profound effects on the person misrecognized.

This story illustrates several core tenets of deaf sociality in Nepal. First, deaf people are responsible for taking care of each other, even from a young age. Second, through appropriate communication and mentorship, people can learn and change. (The correlate of this theory is that deaf people who cease to spend time with other deaf people wither socially and intellectually, and indeed one of the participants in the Old Deaf Project, who had attended the Naxal school in its early days but then stopped, was described to me once as such.) Third, deaf people can provide communication and mentorship to other deaf people in ways that hearing people cannot or do not, and in doing so they can make significant interventions in their lives. Although Prajwal did not say so directly, the implication was that Prajwal—himself a young child—was able to teach his friend fundamental skills that the friend's own family could not or did not.[25]

The following excerpt from my fieldnotes also paints a portrait of deaf people as responsible for and capable of socializing other deaf people in very basic ways. In a conversation with Pashu Dhital, a deaf activist and leader, he suggested that as part of my research, I might help him in his desire to

> document how to change poor, uneducated deaf people. He described how you find deaf people in these villages, and they're dirty and their clothes are torn and they don't know how to eat properly or take care of themselves, and first you teach them how to be clean and how to eat. And how to sign, I added. Yes, he said. He said he wants to film this for 25–30 minutes every day, from that first dirty state to the last day (at the end of a couple months), when they would sign for themselves. And this would show how deaf people can be transformed through education and care.[26]

In Pashu's initial description of what he wanted me to document, he did not focus on deaf villagers' communicative skills; rather, he highlighted the deaf villagers' failure to care for themselves and implicitly the failure of their families to care for them. The ability or act of caring for one's bodily self is attributed not to the innate capacities of an individual but to a self properly enmeshed with others.

There are important parallels and differences here between NSL signers' theories of socialization and academic theories of language deprivation and acquisition as discussed in the introduction. Both emphasize the critical role that signing with others plays in deaf children's development. In academic explications the emphasis has generally been on accessible *language*, though interaction is also framed as important. In NSL signers' socialization theories, as the rest of this chapter demonstrates, the emphasis is on accessible *interaction*, whether that interaction is in NSL or natural sign, although it is clear that NSL signers also consider the differences between them to matter. Hoffmann-Dilloway (2016:72–75) makes a similar point, comparing the very different communicative practices of Nepali deaf people whom she calls "homesigners" who were raised in settings with fewer or more opportunities to engage in "communicative interaction with willing participants."

These examples show that deaf NSL signers view sociality as going far beyond communication and yet depending on it as well; communicative sociality, in other words, is both "about" communication but also critical for other kinds of relationality. Neither Pashu nor Prajwal suggested that deaf people should bathe or feed each other, but that as capable deaf people, they should assume that other deaf people are also capable of such actions, even if they are not currently performing them, and they should teach them how to do so. Critically, NSL does not appear strictly necessary to such endeavors. Pashu makes it clear that the first order of business would be to teach deaf persons to take care of their own bodies; this teaching would involve communicating, and that communication by definition would be natural sign, not NSL. Similarly, Prajwal first would have endeavored to engage with his friend in whatever way he could. In other words, what makes deaf NSL signers able to communicate with deaf non-NSL signers is natural sign and their willingness to engage beyond conventional language.

Yet recall that both Sagar and Furba described natural sign as a communicative mode used by, and even learned from, hearing people. If not only deaf NSL signers but also hearing people (can) use natural sign, then why have these deaf people not already been taught to care for themselves? An interview with a deaf leader, Rajan Khadgi, about KAD's efforts to establish the Old Deaf Project offers a poignant answer to this question. At first Rajan explains that old deaf people don't understand NSL but do understand natural sign, which he defines as "[what is used in] their homes with their families," implying that hearing family members and old deaf people can communicate. Soon after, however, Rajan says this: "At home, hearing family members enjoy themselves, but old deaf people don't. They can't understand or communicate; they have to sit there passively. It's as if they're fools, SUPPRESSED and sad. Thus the idea was that if KAD opened a program for old deaf, they could participate. They would meet regularly, and their understanding would increase. They would realize they were all deaf. They could SIGN with each other and use NATURAL-SIGN. Their communication would come together. They would enjoy themselves and be happy, and be able to let go of how they felt with their families."[27]

Given the juxtaposition of these two scenes—old deaf people using natural sign with their families; old deaf people sitting alone among their relatives—I take Rajan to be suggesting that in family settings, hearing people frequently, perhaps usually, don't *bother* to communicate with deaf people. This resonates powerfully with what Kushalnagar et al. (2020) describe as "communicative neglect," although their work focuses on deaf people's communicative experiences during childhood. In the examples from Pashu and Prajwal, it is unstated whether the families did not try to teach their deaf members how to care for themselves or whether they were unable to. It is also left implicit how the ability of deaf people to teach them relates both to NSL signers' skill in using natural sign and their willingness to put in the effort to communicate with other deaf people. The complex relationship between willingness to communicate with deaf people and the capacity to do so is central to the following sections and to chapters 4 and 5.

WAYS OF SPEAKING AND SIGNING
ABOUT DEAF PEOPLE

I return now to the word *lāṭo* and to NSL signers' critiques of both the word and the set of assumptions and actions its usage indexes. In doing so, I further flesh out key concepts articulated by NSL signers that are grounded in their individual and collective experiences of contingent communication across NSL and natural sign and that in turn inform my approach to natural sign. Through NSL signers'

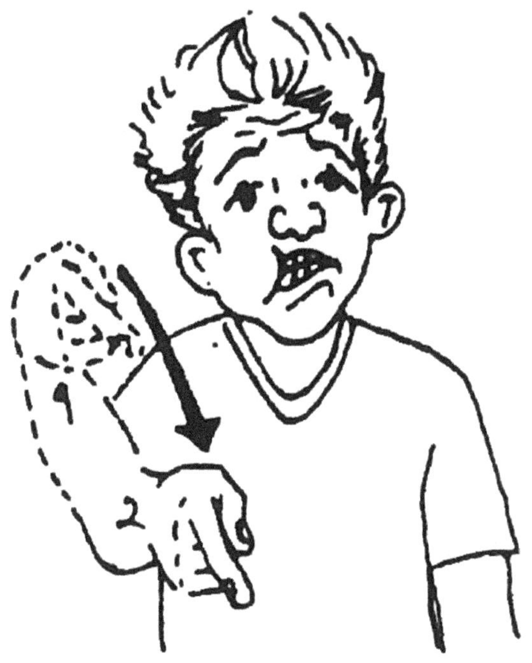

FIGURE 8. The sign that can accompany the mouthing of *lāṭo*. One hand, index finger extended, moves forcefully downward; the signer's facial expression is rueful. Illustration by Pratigya Shakya (NDFN 2003:159). Reproduced by permission from the National Federation of the Deaf Nepal (NDFN).

critique of the word *lāṭo*, I unpack what I mean with the English phrases *situated intelligibility* and *communicative* or *interactional vulnerability*.

Given formal definitions, it is not surprising that NSL signers reject the use of the word to refer to deaf people. One Nepali-English dictionary defines *lāṭo* as "a mute person; a person with a speech impediment," or, in its adjectival form, "foolish, stupid," "numb" (as in a foot that has fallen asleep), or "naive, artless, guileless" (Schmidt 1994). Another defines the nominal as "half-wit; idiot" and the adjectival as "dumb; dull; stupid; inarticulate" (Singh 2004). Neither definition mentions being deaf or unable to hear, though the former does include a sample sentence, the translated version of which reads "The mute have their own language," presumably a reference to deaf people and signed communication.

The word *lāṭo* does not appear in the NSL dictionary that was nearly ubiquitous in NSL signers' homes during my fieldwork (NDFN 2003). In practice, NSL signers express this word with one of the following strategies:

1. they fingerspell it in the NSL manual alphabet, which corresponds to Nepali *devanāgari* script;
2. they fingerspell and mouth *lāṭo*; or
3. they mouth *lāṭo* (without fingerspelling it) while performing the sign in figure 8.

I have the sense that this third strategy functions as quoted speech imputed to hearing people. The sign in this strategy appears in the 2003 dictionary with the

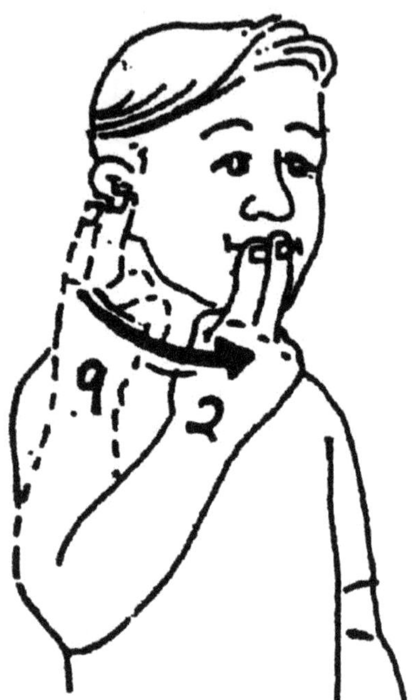

FIGURE 9. The sign DEAF. The index and middle fingers of one hand move from ear to mouth; the signer's facial expression is pleasant. Illustration by Pratigya Shakya (NDFN 2003:17). Reproduced by permission from the National Federation of the Deaf Nepal (NDFN).

gloss *DAMAN* 'SUPPRESSION.' I have only seen it used to accompany the mouthing of *lāṭo*, whereas a second sign glossed SUPPRESSION gets used when talking about suppressive or oppressive actions or situations, as in Rajan's quote about old deaf people.

The NSL sign in figure 9, meanwhile, refers to or describes a deaf person, deaf society, and so forth, and is glossed and translated—in NSL dictionaries, by deaf signers, and by hearing interpreters—with the Nepali *bahirā* and the English *deaf*. A Nepali-English dictionary defines *bahiro*—a version of *bahirā*—simply as "deaf" (adjectival) or "a deaf person" (nominal) (Schmidt 1994). The adjectival example sentence uses *bahiro*, while the nominal example sentence uses *bahirā*. I have seen *bahiro* listed as a derogatory term and *bahirā* as the appropriate term, so I use only the latter unless quoting.

The word *lāṭo* has as much or more to do with other people's (perceptions of) someone's intelligence as with that person's perceived inability—whether permanent or temporary—to hear or speak. It is also true that dictionary definitions are not necessarily indicative of vernacular expression, and thus it might be argued that when people say *lāṭo* to talk about someone who is deaf, they do not necessarily mean everything conveyed by the word *lāṭo*. One young man in Dhankuta told me that the word was simply an aspect of "our colloquial speech" (*hāmro ṭhet bhāshā/boli*), implying that villagers' use of the word was not intended offensively.[28] At the same time, when I was living in Maunabudhuk, where the word was widely used, I noticed that family members of deaf people often—though not always—referred to their loved ones using different terms, such as *apānga* 'disabled.' Moreover, a common refrain that a given deaf person doesn't seem *lāṭo* or even *bahirā* offers evidence that the derogatory shades of meaning in *lāṭo* are always present, not only in the word itself but also in the expectations sutured to the figure of a deaf person.

In 2002, when I first spent time with deaf people in Nepal, I noticed that hearing people frequently expressed surprise when they failed to recognize someone as deaf. In the years since, I have heard hearing Nepalis from a variety of regional, class, and *jāt* 'caste/ethnic' backgrounds remark countless times that a deaf person "does not seem deaf." I use the English here to cover a range of Nepali phrases, including "*lāṭo jasto chhaina* 'isn't like a *lāṭo* person,'" "*boldaina/ sundaina jasto dekhidaina* 'doesn't look like someone who can't speak/hear,'" and "*sunne jastāi rahechha* 'surprisingly or contrary to the speaker's expectation, just like a hearing person.'" I have unintentionally elicited such comments by showing hearing friends photographs of deaf friends, such as in the days before smartphones, when perusing photo albums and stacks of photos was a common activity, and I often responded with indignance. I want to hold onto that indignance as part of my own interpellation into deaf sociality and ethics, as well as to think about what such statements reveal about hearing sociality. I suggest that they indicate a hearing person's recognition of dissonance between their idea of what deaf people look/are like and the way they perceive the person or people in the photograph. In other words, such statements indicate that the token has deviated from the hearing person's imagined type—one might say these are instances of someone's recognition of their misrecognition, to invoke Graif (2018).

During my fieldwork, Ganga Limbu was in his thirties, a member of the local government in Maunabudhuk, and a good friend to both Sagar and me. He once told me a story about the first time he met Sagar. When they were introduced, Ganga was told that Sagar was a teacher but didn't get a chance to talk with him, so Ganga found him later that day. Not knowing he was deaf, Ganga spoke to Sagar and then kept speaking, but Sagar didn't reply. Feeling shy, and wondering "*kasto kālko māsṭar* 'what kind of a teacher [is this person]'?," Ganga stopped talking. When I asked if Sagar hadn't explained that he couldn't hear, Ganga replied that he had done so only later, because the whole time Ganga was talking, Sagar had been facing the other direction.[29]

This story disarmingly pokes fun at Ganga's own confusion while revealing that at least back when he first met Sagar, Ganga was unlikely to think of a teacher as anything other than hearing. Moreover, nothing about Sagar's visual appearance, other than his refusal to turn around, contradicted Ganga's presuppositions about the category of *teacher*. To draw on Liechty's (2003:143–144) analysis of how Nepalis easily identify the "embodied features" or, citing Bourdieu (1977), "bodily *hexis*" that reveal where people are from, their caste, their educational background, and so forth, Sagar's bodily hexis—including his posture and clothing—must have differed from the deaf people with whom Ganga was familiar or from his image of deaf people. Unlike the deaf adults Ganga knew in Maunabudhuk (most of whom had not gone to school), Sagar grew up going to a residential deaf school. He also had spent a lot of time in urban centers and dressed in the latest fashions of his age group. Thinking about this again at a remove of over a decade, what strikes me is that the person who introduced Sagar likely would have mentioned that he was a teacher of deaf people (however this was phrased in Nepali), which would have made the category *deaf* present in the conversation. And even so, Ganga thought that Sagar heard him but strikingly chose not to respond.

Relatedly, a teacher in Maunabudhuk told me that before meeting Sagar, he thought that you could always tell if someone was deaf from the way they walk, their facial expressions, and their hand movements (the latter, I assume, even when not signing, as Sagar of course signed), but that Sagar walked and looked "just like us, like speaking people."[30] Although hearing people in this area do differentiate among deaf residents (discussed in chapter 2), these comments are evidence that the figure of a deaf person is somewhat monolithic. Indeed the social typification of what deaf people are like is so entrenched that even people in Maunabudhuk who knew Sagar well would sometimes ask, "But he can hear, can't he? He just can't speak?" Once, memorably, a woman with whom Sagar chatted and joked almost daily requested that he stick out his tongue for inspection, searching for a bodily fact to which his seeming difference—not from her but from other deaf people—might adhere or that might explain the dissonance she felt between her image of deaf people and her experience of Sagar as a deaf person.

CRITIQUING THE SOCIAL CONSTRUCTION OF UNINTELLIGIBILITY

When deaf people decry the use of *lāṭo*, they are protesting the derogatory meanings conveyed by the word itself as well as the deeply held assumptions about deaf people indexed by the above stories. An examination of publicly articulated statements against the word reveals that this protest employs two primary rhetorical strategies—namely, equating speech and sign as forms of communication and listing the positive attributes of deaf people to contradict the pejorative attributes implicit in *lāṭo*. Moreover, this protest is a call for hearing people to treat deaf people differently than they often do.

At the 2009 NDFN General Assembly, Rajendra Sharma, a longtime deaf leader from Pokhara, recalled the history of the deaf movement in Nepal: "I am very happy because [the result of deaf organizing and activism is that] our communication is good. Just as hearing people have their speech, we deaf people have our sign. Speech and sign are equal. There should be a moratorium on the word *lāṭo* [fingerspelled]. Just because hearing people speak, this doesn't make us deaf people fools—our bodies are fine, we can walk, we can do work, help people, so we are actually equal."[31] Before he even mentions the word *lāṭo*, Rajendra posits a relationship of equivalence: hearing is to speech as deaf is to sign. In other words, what matters is not *how* someone communicates but *that* they communicate. Rajendra then articulates a theory that different human capacities—bodily, mental, communicative, moral, economic—are separable. Deaf people are physically unimpaired ("our bodies are fine, we can walk"), capable of productive labor ("we can do work"), and situated within networks of sociality ("we can help people," reminiscent of Dawa Gurung's comment in the introduction), just like hearing people. The emphasis on deaf people being productive, able to walk, and so forth might seem like a distancing tactic from other disabilities; however, I interpret it more as a call for nondisabled people not to misrecognize or equate different kinds of disabilities. The core traits Rajendra mentions of course represent only one of many possible understandings of what constitutes personhood within Nepal across time and space (e.g., McHugh 1989; Desjarlais 1992; Leve 1999; Pradhan 2020).

At the same program, Raghav Bir Joshi, a former president of the NDFN and the only deaf member of the first Constituent Assembly (now dissolved), made a similar argument, inflected with his signature humor and insight: "Hearing people think that deaf people are fools, but this is not the case. Our minds are still fine. We can't speak or hear, but our minds and our hands and our signing are good. Hearing people's way of thinking is oppressive. Let me make an analogy. Let's say there's a car. The horn is broken, it can't produce a sound, but the rest of the car is in great condition. Would we throw away the whole car? Those people [with oppressive attitudes] should think about that!"[32] Raghav makes two points here with the analogy. First, like Rajendra, he points out that although deaf people don't necessarily use sounds to do so, they are perfectly capable of communicating. Second, Raghav suggests that when members of hearing society treat deaf people as if they were "fools," they are in fact "throwing away" a valuable resource in "great condition." The unstated, and very funny, takeaway is that the *real* fool is someone who throws away an entire car because of a broken horn—in a country where most people, if they own a vehicle at all, have a motorcycle or scooter.

At the farewell program in Maunabudhuk, Sagar's speech took a similar tack, not surprising in that he had attended the General Assembly where the above speeches were given, as well as other NDFN-sponsored programs. Indeed the iterative quality of the speeches at the General Assembly and the appearance of similar rhetoric in other contexts exemplify how national events serve as nodes for the circulation of particular deaf rhetorics and logics. This is what Sagar said, using fingerspelling to articulate *lāṭo*: "To look down on and consider deaf people *lāṭo* is unacceptable. *BAHIRĀ* must be said. Look at the deaf people here in front of us: they are clean, they are capable, they are not *lāṭo*. You can see this for yourselves. They are thoughtful and capable of walking in a straight line. They do not gesticulate randomly. They are not intellectually disabled, that's different. They are deaf."[33]

Like the older leaders quoted above, Sagar points out the positive traits of deaf people, including their cleanliness. He further specifies what deaf people are *not*: people whose moving hands mean nothing, people who are intellectually disabled. While it might be argued that the 2009 NDFN speeches are referring to NSL signers (and not necessarily all deaf Nepalis), Sagar explicitly frames his comments as about the deaf people "here in front of us," all of whom were natural signers, albeit natural signers who had taken an NSL class. The implicit accusation in these utterances is that when deaf people move their hands (whether to produce NSL or natural sign), it is *hearing people* who fail to understand that they are saying something meaningful. Indeed Raghav Bir Joshi made this explicit and took the observation to its logical end. Here he articulates *lāṭo* by mouthing it and using the sign in figure 8: "If we deaf are *lāṭo* because we can't understand hearing people with their sweet talk, then hearing people who can't understand deaf signing are equally *lāṭo*."[34]

Acharya (1997) invokes a similar premise: "The derogatory term *lāṭo* is used to describe the deaf in Nepali society. However, in a situation in which a conversation is ongoing between deaf signers, a hearing onlooker who does not know sign language is him/herself *lāṭo*."[35] In this written version (implied but not explicitly stated in Raghav's), deaf signers signing *with each other* are revealed not to be *lāṭo*; they—if not the hearing people who watch them—understand each other just fine. The "hearing people can be *lāṭo*" trope thus insists that who is *lāṭo* is contextual and not tied to deafness or signing per se. Relatedly, the importance of deaf society is not only in the use of NSL but also in how it makes possible the configuration of multiple signers communicating together. And NSL signers are not the only ones to draw this conclusion. Once, while I was talking with a group of older hearing men at a teashop in Maunabudhuk, one of them—who would not have encountered this joke in NSL or in writing—stated that when deaf people sign, it is the hearing who become *lāṭo*. It is doubtful that he was strictly differentiating between a group of NSL signers and a group of natural signers; what matters is that when deaf people communicate with each other, they are revealed as not being unintelligible after all. On the contrary, it is hearing people who become *lāṭo*. In the same vein, Graif (2018: 121) writes in relation to a deaf protester's reflections on the importance of NSL signers signing together in public that "the sight of an exuberant crowd signing in unison serves to displace the category of deafness away from generalized encounters with *lāṭohood* and onto the fact of a self-engaged deaf community."

While in some senses the negative connotations of *lāṭo* focus on deaf people as not speaking, or not speaking clearly, in these formulations, hearing people are *lāṭo* not because they fail to *produce* (what are recognized by others as) communicative forms but because they fail to *understand* the forms that others have produced. Critically, the (in)ability to understand—and to be understood—is contingent on who is speaking/signing and who is listening/watching. In other words, being *lāṭo* is not an inherent, essential, or fixed attribute but rather relational and dependent on context.

COMMUNICATIVE AND INTERACTIONAL VULNERABILITY

Yet the trope's ironic humor—hearing people can be *lāṭo* too!—rests on the fact that while in theory anyone can be rendered unintelligible (i.e., anyone can not-understand and be not-understood), in practice it is much more likely to happen to deaf people compared to hearing people. The hearing *lāṭo* joke thus invokes a theory of situated intelligibility, which both legitimates deaf people *and* acknowledges their communicative and interactional vulnerability. This vulnerability helps to account for an ambiguity I detected between an argument that deaf people are categorically not *lāṭo* and an argument that only certain kinds of deaf people are not *lāṭo*. A hearing teacher of the deaf addressed the mostly-hearing audience at the end of Maunabudhuk's NSL program with the following words, exemplifying this ambiguity:

> In this six-month program, the reason for providing the deaf with sign language [*sānketik bhāshā*]—that is to say, what is in their own hearts, their emotions, to express these, they will have been using only their natural language [*prakritik bhāshā*]. Now in these modern times, they also have a "mother language" [*mātribhāshā*], that is, for the deaf, sign language is their "mother language." And a program such as this one, its reason is so that they can express what is in their hearts, their emotions, and make others understand. What is more, it seems to us—in village homes, we continue to say *lāṭālāṭi*, of incompetent people [*najanna*], people who don't understand [*nabujhna*], foolish people [*agyānta*]. Saying *lāṭālāṭi* is unacceptable; when speaking of *bahirā*, we must say *bahirā*. Because calling people who understand *lāṭālāṭi*, well, that's not right, to say this to/of uncomprehending people, well, that's okay.[36]

Like Rajendra and others, the teacher here enters a discussion of *lāṭo* through a discussion of sign language and, like NSL signers, explicitly contrasts "natural language" (i.e., natural sign), with "sign language" (i.e., NSL). Moreover, he sets up a line of demarcation that places deaf people qua deaf people safely on the non-*lāṭo* side but leaves room for the possibility that there are people of whom it is *thikāi* 'okay, more or less alright' to say *lāṭo*. It is unclear whether he means that it is okay because as *nabujhne* (uncomprehending) people, they *are* in fact *lāṭo* or because as *nabujhne* people they will not understand, and thus not be hurt by, the word.[37]

While it might be easy to dismiss these words as a hearing person's problematic musings, I once saw a deaf NSL signer say explicitly that there are *lāṭo* deaf people. In a discussion between two young deaf women, Gita, who had more formal education, asked Sushila if she wanted to continue her studies. Sushila said yes, but that she was too old to do so, and proceeded to describe how as a girl she had attended a hearing school. She made one friend but had trouble understanding the teacher, and the other students made fun of her for not being able to hear or speak. Later, after dropping out, she learned NSL, and the people who had teased her apologized. Gita responded to Sushila's story by saying that she should not be sad and should keep trying to further herself. She then relayed a parallel story, revealing that she used to be called *lāṭo* (which she fingerspelled), but later the people who had said this realized they were wrong. She added, "These days there are many *bahirā*, but few *lāṭo*. There are *lāṭo* in the villages, but there are so many deaf schools now in different places."[38]

In both Sushila's and Gita's stories, hearing people taunt the deaf protagonist, only to realize the error of their ways. In Sushila's recounting, this realization is explicitly linked to her acquisition of NSL. That is, Sushila frames the change in hearing people's attitude toward her in terms of a transformation in her own communicative capacities. By becoming someone who could easily understand and be understood by others (NSL signers if not hearing teachers), she created the conditions of possibility for hearing people to recognize that she could communicate even if she couldn't hear or speak. Gita, meanwhile, did not specify the temporal relationship between her own linguistic competence—she learned NSL relatively young—and hearing people's realization that calling her *lāṭo* was wrong. In fact, her final comment suggests that as a deaf person educated from a young age, she never fit into the *lāṭo* category. Yet in firmly staking her claim to being *bahirā*, she explicitly says that there are deaf people who belong in the *lāṭo* category. In Gita's formulation, then, the categories of *bahirā* and *lāṭo* are distinctive and mutually exclusive, separated by space, by education, and by communicative practice.

Recall that Rajendra Sharma, quoted earlier, situated the equality of sign and speech in relation to the growth of deaf organizations and social networks. Stating that deaf and hearing people "are actually equal," he too noted that things are different in villages. He said: "There is one place left, the village, where the word *lāṭo* is still used, where the culture continues, but we hope that with our efforts this will change in the future."[39] In fact, people in cities also use the word *lāṭo*, and I am not claiming that Rajendra thinks it is appropriate to call deaf villagers *lāṭo*. But what then is he suggesting? Prior to this moment, Rajendra has given an account of deaf Nepalis' history, praised deaf signing, and named signed communication (and other capabilities) as evidence that deaf people are not *lāṭo*. Given the context, it is clear that when Rajendra refers to signing, he means Nepali Sign Language, and deaf villagers as a category do not sign NSL. I wonder, therefore, whether the "culture" to which Rajendra refers consists entirely of hearing people's lack of proper understanding of deaf people's capacities or whether it also includes deaf villagers' lack of NSL. His framing of the issue suggests the stakes for NSL signers both of NSL itself and of participating in a form of communicative sociality in which they are consistently intelligible.

At the same time, deaf Nepalis' discourses more generally emphasize that anyone can be rendered *lāṭo* and that communication in natural sign is absolutely possible. While decrying the word *lāṭo*, moments like this hint that some deaf people might correctly (in the semantic, not moral sense) be called *lāṭo* because they are not intelligible in the way that NSL signers are. The "hearing *lāṭo*" joke reveals that intelligibility is contingent on social factors, and NSL signers view learning NSL and participating in deaf society as the best way to ensure that they are not treated as *lāṭo*. Yet a slight variation on the above joke shows that deaf NSL signers also recognize themselves as vulnerable to being ignored or not understood, certainly in comparison to hearing people.

At the 2009 NDFN program, Ramesh Shrestha, a deaf leader and teacher, characterized deaf people's historical relationship with the Nepali state: "In the past the Nepali government did not treat deaf people as equal to hearing people. We explained our plight, told them we had no sign language training, requested their assistance. Yet even though we told them this repeatedly, they paid no attention [literally, they did not hear us], because they did not understand our signing. And I ask, if you can't hear us sign, who is deaf? We or you?" In asking these questions, Ramesh uses the standard NSL sign DEAF (as in figure 9), while mouthing *bahirā*. By calling the government "deaf" and asking why they were unable to "hear" their signs, Ramesh neatly plays on the literal and figurative meanings of *deaf* and *hearing*.[40] Yet with this same rhetorical device he also implies that the experience of being unable to understand, of being outside shared language practices and incapable of making sense of what others say (as the government was in relation to deaf signing), belongs not only to *lāṭo* people but to *bahirā* ones as well. The strict separation of *bahirā* people from *lāṭo* people shows slippage, unintelligibility being a state to which *all* deaf people are vulnerable, precisely because intelligibility is—as deaf discourse so powerfully demonstrates—a socially produced, relational quality.

The *Students' Companion Dictionary* (Singh 2004) in fact offers this definition of *bahiro* [*sic*]: "deaf; hard of hearing; inattentive." While *deaf* and *hard of hearing* are in and of themselves neutral adjectives, the word *inattentive* reveals a collapse in the dictionary writer's perspective between a person not being able to hear someone and not paying attention to them, a collapse between an inability and an unwillingness to attend to someone. It is the same collapse, but inverted, that NSL signers highlight and critique when they argue that hearing people should (and can) communicate with deaf people but often do not. Sagar described different ways that hearing people treat deaf people in a speech at the end of the Maunabudhuk NSL program for which he was the teacher.

> In the villages [deaf people] are made to sit like donkeys, doing nothing but work. This is not necessary. Deaf and hearing are equal! Deaf people are oppressed, while hearing people travel to foreign countries, but we should be treated equally. Property should be divided equally [between deaf and hearing heirs]. Making deaf people stay at home, oppressed, while hearing people are allowed to *GHUMNA* 'WANDER-AROUND' is unacceptable. Deaf and hearing are equal. . . . Hiring a deaf person but paying only a pittance for their labor is also unacceptable. Their guardians should advise them on this as well, for their guardians to be passive is unacceptable. To shoo deaf people away from stores is unacceptable. To tell a deaf person repeatedly, "Just a second," and keep talking with other hearing people is unacceptable. Shopkeepers should talk with deaf and hearing people in turn.[41]

Sagar creates a striking contrast between actions that oppress, such as not paying deaf people fairly or shooing them away from stores, and actions that create and affirm equality, such as paying them enough or talking with them in turn. He juxtaposes quantifiable, even legally inflected ethical demands—fair wages and inheritances—with the ethical demands of everyday life. Families, he tells the primarily hearing audience, should expect all members to shoulder equal shares of work; parents of deaf people should teach their children to stand up for themselves and should stand up for them when necessary; shopkeepers should talk with deaf and hearing customers in turn.

In contrast to the wish expressed by deaf people that in the future all hearing people would learn Indian Sign Language (Friedner 2015:157–161), Sagar is firmly focused on the possibilities of the present. As mentioned in the introduction, attending to such calls might be thought of as an anthropology of the *meanwhile*. Not only *should* deaf and hearing people enter into communicative relationships, they *can*, right now, so long as hearing people are willing to do so. Knowing NSL and being around other NSL signers is the surest guarantee that deaf people can participate in communicative sociality, but said participation does not have to depend on knowing NSL or even on being part of deaf society. If deaf society is a social space in which deaf people ethically orient toward communicating with each other in sign, whether NSL or natural sign, Sagar's call is for society writ large to also be a space in which the possibilities of communicating with deaf people are felt as ethical demands. This call, and its fulfillment, are possible because natural sign exists, and yet the very fact that Sagar articulates it points to deaf signers' interactional vulnerability.

CONCLUSION

NSL signers' discourse makes clear that to be deaf is not to be *lāṭo* in a permanent or ontological sense; but to be deaf when others are unable or unwilling to sign with you is to be treated as if you were *lāṭo*; and to be treated by others as if you were *lāṭo* positions you in that moment as *being lāṭo*. Thus deaf Nepalis' critiques of and campaign against the word *lāṭo* are not only a protest against being *perceived* as *lāṭo* but also against being *made lāṭo*. They reveal both the distinctions and the connections between communicative differences, "sensory asymmetries" and "sensory politics" (De Meulder et al. 2019), and communicative or inter-actional vulnerability. On the one hand, NSL signers' lived daily practices and discourse forcefully dismantle the assumption that to be deaf is to have difficulty communicating. They embody and objectify NSL as both the medium and the result of socially, politically, and personally meaningful interactions among deaf people. On the other hand, NSL signers also know, and in their discourse rec-ognize, that being deaf makes them vulnerable during interactions with hearing people who assume them to be *lāṭo*.

The categories and logics explored in this chapter, the ones I learned by spend-ing time in deaf society with NSL signers, have helped to guide the fundamentally relational approach to natural sign that I take throughout this book. They reveal that conventional language is both critically important and not always necessary; that to be deaf is not to be *lāṭo* but to be deaf makes it more likely that hearing people will treat you as *lāṭo*; that knowing NSL and other NSL signers makes it less likely that you will experience being made *lāṭo*, in part because NSL signers acquire linguistic skills that affect the effectiveness of their natural sign use, and in part because NSL signers get to spend more time engaging in communicative sociality with other NSL signers and less with hearing people; and that being an NSL signer does not protect you fully. If hearing people ignore, misunderstand, or even try but nevertheless fail to make sense of deaf signers, deaf signers often have little recourse, precisely because to protest or resolve such treatment would require that hearing people pay attention to and understand them in the first place. NSL signers, especially those in urban areas, can gaze beyond any given conversation in which they are treated as *lāṭo*: to their next conversation in NSL; to growing recognition by hearing people that NSL is a language, even if not one they know; to increasing availability of trained NSL-Nepali interpreters. Natural signers cannot.

The remainder of this book enters more fully into the worlds of natural signers, and into the possibilities, limits, and ethics of natural sign communication beyond NSL networks. Natural sign, almost by definition, involves a great deal of variation, and I ground my discussion of it in a particular time and place: Maunabudhuk and Bodhe in 2010 (and into the present). The specific setting of these villages shapes what natural signing is like there. At the same time, my work and travel elsewhere in Nepal and indeed the very naming and characterizing of the phenomenon by NSL signers suggests that natural sign is an important dimension of many, almost certainly most, deaf Nepalis' experiences.

2

———

Taxonomic Urges

In May 2010, Sagar Karki and I were standing in the courtyard between a house and an open-air blacksmithery on the far side of Bodhe, a good hour's walk from the bazaar in Maunabudhuk, where we both lived and where Sagar was teaching an NSL outreach class for deaf adults. One of Sagar's responsibilities was to facilitate the enrollment of deaf children into one of the district's three residential classes for deaf students, and we had been following the trail of a young deaf girl whom we had been told was of school age. An acquaintance directed us to a small jeweler's shop located by the football field at one end of Maunabudhuk's bazaar; the man we met there suggested we go to the school in Bodhe; and the teachers at the school asked a cousin of the family in question to guide us along the paths from the school to the house. Upon arrival, we met the young girl's grandparents and several other relatives including her uncle, who was around Sagar's age, though not the girl herself or her mother, who were visiting the latter's *māitighar* 'natal home.'

As we talked, the grandfather paused from the task of fixing a tool, for which another man sat waiting. In Nepali and NSL (I served as translator) we discussed the possibility of the girl attending a deaf residential class. The family seemed open to the idea, although over the next couple months they decided that she was too young to send so far away and that they would wait another year or two. During our discussion we asked if they knew any other deaf people in the area; they said no. Then toward the end of the conversation, one of the family members remembered that in fact, as I wrote in my fieldnotes, "the man sitting right there [waiting for his tool to be fixed] is also 'like that.'" I continued:

> We turned to him and he kind of grinned at us and Sagar and I talked to him, he speaks pretty much fluently but is definitely hard of hearing, and proclaimed [to have] no interest in going to school [i.e., attending the NSL class] and didn't want to take us to his house because he had to go cut grass [for fodder] first. He wasn't at all unfriendly, just very sure of where his priorities were. The [girl's] family members said that we should talk to his mother, because what she says rules, so we decided to go find the house, especially since they also said that his wife is also "like that," and even more so (i.e., hears/speaks less). A young boy led us most of the way there, and then we asked at the house above theirs, where they said there were actually three deaf/hard of hearing people, the mother too.

My fieldnotes go on to explain that upon meeting her, I perceived the mother as someone who had been hearing most of her life and was becoming deaf in old age.[1]

One of the key ways that scholars have approached deaf sociality and communication—particularly in settings beyond large, urban, institutionally scaffolded, and/or nationally scaled communities—involves the enumeration of deaf people in terms of numbers, familial relationships, and overall percentage of some sociospatially delineated population, such as a village. These figures stand in, implicitly or explicitly, for the likelihood that a deaf person can regularly engage in social interactions in sign. While this book argues that ethical orientations regarding deaf people and signing are not reducible to numbers or even familiarity, it also is evident that demographics and relationships very much matter. Indeed, part of what is striking about Maunabudhuk and Bodhe is that in terms of deaf people as a percentage of the total population, these villages resemble some of the settings where shared sign languages have developed. A more detailed analysis, however, reveals consequentially different demographic and communicative patterns. These differences and patterns are the focus of the second half of this chapter, where I explore what makes Maunabudhuk and Bodhe distinct from the classic descriptions and models of places where both deaf and hearing people sign. I argue that this distinction demands a rethinking of deaf persons and signing as an integral part of human histories and presents across space and time.

It would be possible to dive immediately into an enumeration of Maunabudhuk and Bodhe's deaf population and a comparison of local natural sign practices in these places to (how scholars classify and describe) other signing practices in other places. Doing so, however, would erase the complexity of the category *deaf*. The particulars of this chapter's opening vignette—the fact that the family seemed to forget about a deaf man "sitting right there," their characterization of the man and his wife as "like that," their assertion in comparison with the neighbor's mention of three deaf people, my own clumsy attempts to describe in written English my and others' observations of people's different relationships to hearing and speech—point to the various ways in which people get perceived, identified, and counted as *deaf*. The vignette offers a sense of the complexities involved in asking and answering questions like the following, whether in the field or in this book: Who is deaf? Who counts as deaf (and who counts them)? What does deaf mean in such accountings?

The first half of this chapter therefore focuses on the social (re)production of the category *deaf*—or rather, the category that in this book I refer to with the English word *deaf*. I consider how deaf residents of Maunabudhuk and Bodhe discuss being deaf. This was not a frequent topic of conversation. As with "culture" more generally, what being deaf means to people was most explicitly articulated in contexts of "interaction" and "confrontation" (Trawick 1990:90) between distinct domains or logics: here, in conversations and lessons in the NSL class about the NSL sign DEAF. These conversations enabled me to get a sense of how deaf residents recognized and constituted themselves as similar and also made distinctions among themselves, particularly in relation to speech and hearing. Next I explore hearing residents' ways of categorizing and counting deaf people in conversations and lists. These sections argue for the importance of ethnographic attention to the socioculturally specific ways that people (get) count(ed) as deaf as well as to the interplay of hearing and deafness, speech and sign, in deaf people's lives and communicative practices (Bahan 2009, 2010; Friedner and Helmreich 2012; Lucas et al. 2015; Kusters 2019; Sanchez 2020; Friedner 2022).

I show that the category *deaf*—itself an imperfect translation of the categories present and (sometimes) named in the field—encompasses a variety of people, including people who use sign exclusively, people who use both speech and sign as primary communicative modalities, and perhaps even a few people who can hear. Deaf studies scholars have long argued that in deaf-centered communities, *deaf* is a social category that goes far beyond audiological status (Padden and Humphries 1988; Ladd 2003). In conversation with scholars including Kusters (2015), Haviland (2016), Hou (2016, 2020), and Goico (2019), this section shows that *deaf* is a culturally specific, socially produced category in hearing-majority communities as well. Moreover, even the question of whether someone hears is more complicated than it might appear.

The second half of this chapter explores the scholarly urge to taxonomize settings and signing, an urge I both resist and yield to. In recent years, as part of a broader proliferation in research on deaf sociality and signed communicative practices, the English-language scholarly literature has manifested a dazzling array of categories used to make sense of the many sociolinguistic circumstances in which deaf people live and communicate and the kinds of signed communication they create and inherit (Nonaka 2007; Green 2014c; Kusters and Hou 2020; Hou and de Vos 2022; Goico and Horton 2023; Moriarty and Hou 2023). The sociolinguistic circumstances in which people use sign are extraordinarily diverse, generally unaccounted for by spoken language–based models, and undeniably give rise to communicative practices that differ both formally and functionally (Hou and de Vos [2022] and Kusters and Lucas [2022] offer related arguments). Classificatory schemas do the important work of both making distinctions and linking similar cases. The taxonomic urge represents important intellectual (and political) impulses toward recognition of both differences and similarities. Yet in the quest to categorize, it can also ignore and erase specificity that matters, or differences that make a difference, to use a common anthropological phrase. Relatedly, scholars often laminate the classification of communicative communities onto the classification of signing (Kisch 2008), even though different kinds of signing practices can appear in apparently similar settings and vice versa.

Contemporary classifications run along two primary axes: sociospatial and temporal. In relation to space, some of the most prominent categories, and ones that are particularly relevant to this discussion, include *home sign* (often written *homesign*), generally understood as the signing of an individual (e.g., Kegl, Senghas, and Coppola 1999), and *shared sign languages* (Nyst 2012, adapting a term from Kisch 2008, cited in Kisch 2012b), generally understood as the signing that emerges in places with a relatively large number of deaf persons across generations. In relation to time, Meir et al. (2010) have distinguished between *emerging sign languages* and *established sign languages*, depending on the age of the language in question. (Appendix 2 further explores the logics underlying these and other categories.)

Some classificatory schemas, or uses of them, involve an implicit or explicit spectrum and/or trajectory of languageness, often moving from gesture to home sign to signed languages (Kusters et al. 2020b; Kusters and Hou 2020). While my approach firmly rejects a single trajectory, it seeks to acknowledge and make further sense of how particular kinds of resources facilitate particular kinds of communication and modes of sociality and vice versa. Moreover, as I argue throughout this book, it is critically important to consider the role of ethical orientations when thinking about relationships among language, communication, interaction, and social settings—relationships that are embedded in more frequently invoked concepts such as critical mass, social proximity, language emergence, and (ease of) understanding.

Although an anthropological cliché, it is also true that I went to the field with one set of categories and returned with another. When writing grants for dissertation fieldwork, I used the term *home sign*, and I continue to find it fruitful to think about natural sign in relation to research on home sign, along with research on shared sign languages and the earlier manifestations of emerging sign languages.[2] However, I have found the primary available categories inadequate to the phenomenon I research, as have other scholars working in other settings (e.g., Hou 2020; Reed 2020, 2022). Thus my use of the terms *natural sign* and *local sign* represents both resistance and acquiescence to the taxonomic urge. As I will show, natural local sign has important features in common with, but also critical differences from, home sign, shared sign languages, and emerging sign languages; so too the places where they are used. These similarities and differences help make sense of the specific characteristics of natural sign discussed in the introduction and previous chapter: its possibilities and precarities, availability and fragility. Indeed, while adding to the taxonomic landscape, I also want to insist that the local concepts and practices with which I work themselves insist on attention to particularity and context.

Finally, I consider how examining what I call *deaf demography* in the context of natural sign pushes against a tendency, even in some work focused on deaf people and signing, to think about the presence of deaf people and signed communication as unusual.[3] This is evident when, for example, deaf people's signs are analyzed as elaborations of hearing people's gestures. There is no doubt that such analyses make sense in certain circumstances; there are locales in which residents can recall when the first deaf person was born within collective memory. Such framings, however, can inadvertently suggest that social time and space are hearing by default. The situation in Maunabudhuk and Bodhe, and indeed Nepal more broadly, requires a radical refiguration of (what is assumed to be) generic space-time. At least in some times and places, the world has always been deaf *and* hearing.

DEAF CONVERSATIONS AND CATEGORIES

In an overview and critique of scholarly literature, Kusters (2010:11, emphasis in original) observes that researchers frequently fail to "report *deaf* people's attitudes and experiences of being deaf" outside of large deaf communities. Building on Kusters, this section centers what deaf people themselves have to say about being deaf. It is important to note, however, that during my fieldwork deaf residents of Maunabudhuk and Bodhe infrequently made reference to their own or others' deafness, whether in sign or a spoken language. The major exception was the conversations analyzed below that happened in the context of Sagar teaching the NSL sign DEAF.

Outside of those conversations, I heard two class participants refer to deaf people with the spoken Nepali word *lāṭo*, a term discussed at length in chapter 1. One of the participants was generally regarded by others and regarded herself as hearing but appeared on a list of potential students and attended class several times because she was interested in the literacy training provided. The other person was socially regarded as deaf; it is impossible for me to say whether her use of the word reflected a negative attitude toward being deaf, and, if so, for what reasons. I wrote in my fieldnotes about two other instances when a deaf person directly mentioned their own or someone else's deafness, these times in sign. Once, Bal Limbu, a deaf man, was complaining about his hearing employer, and Sanu Kumari Limbu, an older deaf woman, told him that "if he's not getting paid [for his work], he shouldn't do the work, and that he was being cheated because he's deaf."[4] This offers evidence that deaf natural signers both perceive and name the ways in which being deaf can render them vulnerable to being taken advantage of by hearing people.

On another occasion, a deaf man from Atharasaya, a village across the valley where Sagar had taught previously, visited Maunabudhuk. Based on notions of deaf sociality and sameness (explored and troubled in Friedner and Kusters 2014), I—and apparently Sagar—expected that the deaf residents would be interested in talking to him, but they were not especially excited to do so. Bal happened to be present, and Sagar tried to get him and the visitor to engage. He told the visitor where Bal lived and that they were both Limbu (pointing to further sameness), but they did not interact very much. At one point, Bal commented, "Neither Sagar nor [this man] can hear or speak, but I can speak." Sagar told Bal that he, Bal, was also deaf, but Bal more or less ignored this statement.[5]

This example illustrates Friedner and Kusters's (2014) argument that a sense of similitude between deaf people is by no means a given and points to how during my fieldwork in Maunabudhuk and Bodhe, deaf and, as shown below, hearing people categorized deaf people together but also differentiated among them on the basis of speech and hearing. This differentiation came into play in the most explicit and elaborate discussions that I witnessed by deaf people about being deaf. A conversation from June 2, about a month and a half into the NSL class, is my first recorded instance of a lesson and ensuing discussion about the NSL sign DEAF (though it is possible that one occurred in the first several weeks the class was running before I moved to Maunabudhuk). I recorded a related conversation on video the following day. Taken together, these conversations reveal the complexities and variations of deaf residents' understandings, definitions, and descriptions of what it is to be deaf, showing that natural signers do not present a blank slate onto which deaf society's logics are inscribed.[6] The issues of translation, (in)commensuration, and (mis)alignment that occur in this mixed NSL–natural sign space also demand recognition of the translation, (in)commensuration, and (mis)alignment that occur between that space and what you are reading in this English-language text.

Here is my description of the first conversation, as I wrote it with pen and paper while sitting in the classroom:

Sagar just taught a brief but powerful (to me anyway) lesson: you are deaf. He explained what [the NSL sign] DEAF meant (not-hearing, not-speaking) and then went around and asked everyone if they are deaf or hearing. Krishna was quick to say he was deaf. Padma was more hesitant, saying he can hear some—he and Bal had just been talking about how they can both hear some, Padma made a high-pitched noise that [to my ear] Bal correctly imitated. But Sagar repeated that Padma is deaf and Padma accepted this and signed DEAF. Bal also at first said he can hear, so Sagar grabbed a small pamphlet laying around and handed it to Bal and instructed him to read it aloud. Sagar then mimed reading Sanskrit scripture at a wedding, and Bal rejected this possibility (whether of the reading, the Sanskritness, or the [possibility that he would be engaged in that kind of activity at a] wedding, I'm not sure) and accepted DEAF. To my surprise Lalita—who [from my perspective] probably has the clearest spoken language production and reception of anyone present today—just signed DEAF when Sagar asked "deaf or hearing?" I signed [the NSL sign] HEARING and Padma and Krishna nodded in approval. [Not of my being hearing per se but of the correctness of the stated facts.] Parvati also said she was deaf, as did Shrila—stating along with an approximation of the sign DEAF that she can't hear. Jyoti first indicated she can talk/hear (which is true) and Sagar did the "read this" routine again, and Jyoti relented (this sounds like it was mean or harsh—the whole time it was playful and light-hearted, as class usually is). Sanu Kumari also said she can talk (true) so Sagar asked if she can talk on a mobile phone (a better test, I thought, than reading aloud). There was some confusion as to whether Sagar was asking whether she *has* a phone, because she kept answering that her son does, and Sagar kept asking, "No, *you*, can *you* talk on a phone?" He showed that he can't, how when he feels his phone ringing he finds a hearing person such as me [to answer it]. Sanu Kumari eventually said she's deaf.

[From my perspective,] there was not a denial of speech or hearing—no pressure to *not* talk but rather a teaching that *despite* (some) speech or hearing, you are deaf. It was an effective lesson. Sagar went around the room again and everyone (except me of course) said they are deaf.[7]

The lesson on the following day, which I recorded on video, began with Sagar asking how many deaf people were present and immediately segued into a brief counting lesson. Then Sagar asked Sanu Kumari whether she was deaf or hearing, and she responded that she could in fact hear and talk, despite, or perhaps not at all in contradiction with, the fact that at the end of the previous day's lesson, she—along with the rest of the class—had seemed to accept Sagar's logic that everyone but me was deaf.

At this point the lesson shifted to defining what the NSL sign DEAF means and teaching people that they *are* deaf. Like the day before, Sagar offered up reading material and then his phone to point out to Sanu Kumari that she could not read aloud or speak on the phone. And like the previous day, Sanu Kumari reacted to him handing her the phone by telling him, "No, that's your phone!" Following a brief adjustment to the angle of the camera and where Sagar stood (this was one of the first classes I filmed), Sagar proclaimed that everyone except me was deaf. He then began to enumerate: "You are deaf, you are deaf, I am deaf," using the NSL sign DEAF. When he got to Buddha Yonjan, however, he clarified: "He's HALF-HEARING, he's HARD-OF-HEARING." (The NSL dictionary [NDFN 2003] glosses both of these signs HARD-OF-HEARING, as per figure 10, but it is helpful to distinguish between them here, especially because HALF-HEARING, literally HEARING-HALF, would most likely be interpretable, whereas HARD-OF-HEARING, an initialized sign at the ear, would be opaque to natural signers.)

Soon after, Sagar asked Sarawata Limbu if she was deaf; Sarawata responded with both speech and sign, indicating that she can hear. Sagar asks her in NSL, "Oh, you're hearing, you speak?" to which Sarawata responds, using the NSL sign SPEAK, "Yes, I speak." Sagar tries to hand Sarawata his phone; she responds in

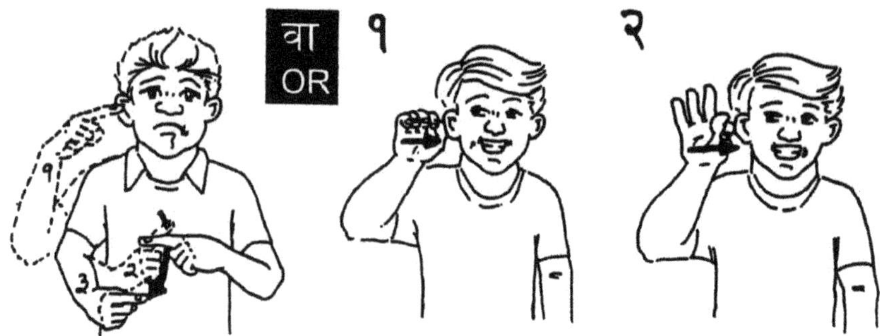

FIGURE 10. NSL signs for HARD-OF-HEARING. On the left, in the sign I gloss HALF-HEARING, a person points with an extended index finger to the ear, then moves the index finger across a second extended finger at chest level to indicate partiality. On the right, in the sign I gloss HARD-OF-HEARING, a person makes two handshapes at the ear, corresponding to the *devanāgari* initials for the Nepali phrase *susta shrawan* 'hard of hearing.' Illustration by Pratigya Shakya (NDFN 2003:17). Reproduced by permission from the National Federation of the Deaf Nepal (NDFN).

natural sign, "My sister-in-law has a phone," to which Krishna Gajmer says, "You can't hear! You're deaf!," using the bivalent sign HEAR and the NSL sign DEAF. The conversation continues, Krishna and Sagar telling Sarawata that she is deaf like them. Sagar, clearly frustrated, asks me to speak with Sarawata. I comply, asking her in Nepali if she can hear. She responds in Limbu, which I don't speak or understand. Later in the conversation Sarawata depicts conversations between herself and her parent(s)-in-law, showing that they use speech as well as sign, and says that she can hear. With her older daughter too, she adds, she uses speech; or perhaps she says that her parents-in-law use speech with her older daughter.

Krishna asks her if she can hear in both ears or only one. Sarawata tells him only one. Krishna replies that he can't hear in either ear, and reports to Sagar that Sarawata can in fact hear in one ear. Sagar responds by saying, "She's deaf! We're all deaf!" He continues: "Can you read [aloud]? Can you talk with your mouth and not use your hands? We sign, we're all deaf." He gives examples of natural signs used in the area, then reiterates: "Hearing people can stand and talk like this with their arms crossed. Deaf people use their hands. Can the two of you, Krishna and Sarawata, speak to each other?" Sarawata replies, "We do speak," then mentions her sister-in-law. Sagar counters by again showing someone signing. The angle of the video makes it hard to see, but it looks like he is acting as if he is using his mouth and signing at the same time. "You're deaf, you sign," he says.

A few minutes later, Sagar returns to the position that "all of us are deaf," thus reincorporating Buddha, whom he had called hard of hearing, back into the category of *deaf* (and ignoring my hearingness). Much later in the conversation, Sagar states that three people present are hard of hearing, one hearing, and seven deaf. This inclusion of the category *hard of hearing* was one of two key differences in relation to the previous day. The second was that on June 3 both Sagar and Sarawata depicted different communicative modalities as an important aspect of defining the sign DEAF and deciding who was deaf, as I explore momentarily.

As with other NSL lessons, Sagar taught the sign DEAF through a combination of NSL signs, natural signs, and bivalent signs. He also offered examples, often using what is known in sign language linguistics as constructed action (Cormier, Smith, and Sehyr 2015) - that is, acting out the role of various characters - and asking his students about their personal experiences. More so than with other lessons, however, teaching the sign DEAF involved complex negotiations, both of its meaning and applicability to specific persons. Some people, such as Krishna, easily agreed that they were deaf, while others, such as Sanu Kumari and Sarawata, repeatedly laid claim to their abilities to speak and to hear. In response, Sagar shifted his definitions and explanations of what the NSL signs DEAF and HEARING mean. For example, early in the conversation on June 3, Sagar equates being hearing with speaking and thus implicitly equates being deaf with not speaking. When Sanu Kumari says she can speak, he moves his focus to whether she can speak on a phone—offering her his own—or read aloud.

As these descriptions make evident, Sagar had a phone, as do many deaf people in Nepal. When Sagar held out his phone to his students, he was asking if they could use it as hearing people do. Hearing villagers also must have been thinking about normatively hearing uses of phones when they asked why Sagar had a phone. In the same vein, I interpret his questions about reading not as a way of disavowing that deaf people can read (he himself could do so) but rather as invoking a shared understanding that deaf people don't usually read aloud using speech (Green 2022b further discusses typification in signing practices). Similarly, although it is unclear from the video if Sagar was watching Sarawata when she depicted herself talking and signing, his shift in emphasis from not hearing or speaking, not using the phone and not reading aloud, to the observation that deaf people must use their hands (implied: even if also speaking), suggests that he was both watching and responding.

These examples also draw attention to the conversational participants' diverse responses and communicative and sensory experiences. Krishna, who seldom if ever used speech and who said he couldn't hear in either ear, quickly understood what the sign DEAF meant and accepted it for himself. Given Sagar's definitions of DEAF as not-speaking and not-hearing, perhaps Krishna experienced the sign with a kind "of course!" feeling, similar to the socially embedded experience of congruence that Kraus (2018) describes for new deaf signers at Gallaudet University. I am not, however, suggesting sensory determinism. Lalita Limbu, who uses speech as much as if not more than Sarawata and who playfully depicted herself talking on the phone by saying, "*ālo, ālo* 'hello, hello,'" said "yes," when asked if she was DEAF. Interestingly, Sagar included Lalita in his list of hard of hearing people, despite her acceptance of the sign DEAF.

Sagar wondered if his repeated claim that Sarawata was deaf made her angry, implying that she did not want to be (seen as) deaf. When Sarawata says to Sagar that she can hear, he seems to interpret this as a rejection of the category *deaf*, which to Sagar indexes an entire world of shared social experiences—in short, what it means to be deaf in deaf society. I take her to mean, much more literally, that she is not deaf in the sense of being a person who can neither hear nor speak—which is how Sagar has just defined the sign. Using the logic of this definition, Sarawata's phenomenological experience of her body and of communication contradict the claim that she is deaf. To be clear, within deaf society there are many people whose sensory and communicative repertoires appear similar to Sarawata's who consider themselves, and are considered by others, to be deaf. In other words, from the perspective of deaf society, Sarawata's experiences are by no means inconsistent with the category *deaf*, but they are inconsistent with Sagar's explicit definition, made succinct for the purposes of pedagogy. In the same vein, when Sagar suggests to Sarawata and Sanu Kumari that they *cannot* hear, I do not think he is trying to deny the validity of their sensory experiences but is instead following the logic of his own definition, which states that a person who is deaf is someone who cannot hear.

Sagar and Sarawata both acknowledge that modality is a key dimension in people's experiences of communicative sociality. Their difference lies in whether not-speaking or using sign is more important. Sarawata, having been told that to be deaf is to not-speak, indicates that she speaks as well as signs. Sagar counters by saying that if someone needs their hands to communicate, they are deaf. They eventually settle their disagreement when Sagar offers Sarawata the option that she is HALF-HEARING, a designation she accepts. It is possible to conclude from this conversation that Sarawata's and Sagar's understandings of DEAF were incommensurable. I suggest, however, that they actually were making different references with the same sign. The NSL sign DEAF was new to Sarawata, so her prior experiences and categories could only be compared with the explicit definition given to her, and not with the broader and more flexible meanings that the sign and category hold for NSL signers. I wonder how Sarawata would have responded if Sagar had originally defined deaf as sign-using rather than not-speaking. It seems worth mentioning here that with the exception of one teenager, who stopped coming to class after some sessions, none of the NSL class attendees expressed confusion, dissatisfaction, or disapproval at having been invited to participate in this deaf, signing space.

Deaf studies has shown that in deaf (sometimes self-identified Deaf) communities, what it is to be deaf or Deaf goes far beyond not-hearing. According to Bauman (2008:12), for example, "two factors combine to form the common ground of a Deaf identity: audiological deafness and use of sign language." The emphasis on "Deaf culture" and on the cultural dimensions of "Deaf identity" makes sense in relation to deaf studies', and deaf people's, battles with biomedical definitions of deafness as lack (Bauman 2008). Yet as Friedner and Helmreich (2012:74) argue, citing Keating and Hadder (2010), "deafness" and "hearing" now "operate as ideal types, which downplays continuums between and multiplicities of sensory capabilities." Works such as "Sensory Orientations" (Bahan 2009, 2010), "Sensations of Sound" (Kolb 2017), a special issue on "deaf and hearing signers' multimodal and translingual practices" (Kusters ed. 2019), "Deafness and Sound" (Sanchez 2020), and "Writing as Being: On the Existential Primacy of Writing for a Deaf Scholar" (Snoddon 2022) indicate a shift away from ideal types and toward acknowledging and exploring deaf peoples' diverse corporeal experiences and communicative practices. Contributing to this shift, I have focused my attention on how participants in the NSL class in Maunabudhuk articulate their own bodily schemas and experiences of signed and spoken communication. In relation to scholarly discussion of entering deaf sociality as a kind of conversion experience (Bechter 2008; Friedner 2014; Kraus 2018), these conversations show that deaf people's definitions of being deaf might not be immediately transparent, relevant, or clear to other deaf people with different social and/or phenomenological experiences.

My analysis also builds on previous scholarship showing that *hearing* as much as *deaf* is a sociocultural category. While prior work has focused on the affects and effects of shifting technologies—from telephones to hearing aids to cochlear implants of various kinds (Mills 2012; Mauldin 2014; Booth 2021; Friedner 2022)—the conversations analyzed here took place in a setting where those particular technologies are not widely utilized for the purposes of medicalizing or measuring people's audiological capacities. Nevertheless, in this setting, hearing—like speaking, not-hearing, and not-speaking—is organized around culturally specific logics and concerns and cannot be understood as portable, transparent, or unmediated descriptions of sensory and communicative configurations and experiences.

MY USE OF THE TERM *DEAF*

In conversation with the growing literature on deaf people's multimodal repertoires and sensoria, I do not in this book distinguish between *deaf* and *hard of hearing* people or experiences, other than when discussing my interlocutors' own distinctions as in the earlier conversations. For me to make these distinctions throughout the book would be untenable for multiple reasons. Lalita, for example, happily acceded to being called both deaf and hard of hearing. Sarawata, meanwhile, seemed to accept the NSL sign HALF-HEARING and to reject the NSL sign DEAF. Yet to refer to her as *hard of hearing* would imply that the English *deaf* and *hard of hearing* and the NSL DEAF and HALF-HEARING are identical. It also would decontextualize her insistence/rejection from the specifics of the conversation and the way Sagar sought to define DEAF. If my goal were to use the terms desired by each of my interlocutors (and if I were writing about named self-identification, that would be a key aim), how would I translate, not only across the complex negotiations of meaning between NSL and natural sign but also into English?

In the spaces where I spent most time—in deaf society, in Maunabudhuk and Bodhe, in homes, and in this classroom—the primary categories in operation are, however imperfectly, best captured by the English words *deaf* and *hearing*. Therefore, when writing about people such as Sagar, Krishna, Sarawata, and Lalita, I use the term *deaf*. I try in this chapter and throughout the book to attend to people's sensory configurations and communicative actions in a way that does not flatten deaf people's experiences—for example, by making explicit the social fact that some of my interlocutors talk with, and talk about talking with, both their mouths and their hands. I remain ambivalent about my decision not to use the phrase *deaf and hard of hearing* in favor of *deaf*, and hope that it will be read in the expansive sense in which it is intended rather than an exclusionary or narrowing one.

HEARING WORDS

In addition to visiting class participants' homes, Sagar and I relied on village-generated lists of deaf people (discussed below) as well as on word-of-mouth (I use the speech-centric phrase on purpose) to seek out and talk to other deaf people in the area. Hearing people in Maunabudhuk and Bodhe refer to a variety of people, including those whom I call *deaf*, with the term *lāṭo*—a Nepali word that connotes someone who has trouble making sense. This word is probably the most common way in spoken Nepali to refer to someone deaf. As much as possible, I refrained from invoking the vernacular *lāṭo* to ask about deaf people, using phrases like *kān nasunne* '[people with] not-hearing ears' or *mukh nabolne* '[people with] not-speaking mouths.' These phrases are by no means unusual ways to talk about deaf people and are examples of a generative Nepali structure in which verb phrases become noun phrases (such as *kām garne mānche* 'work-doing people'—i.e., workers). Nevertheless, it is possible that my use of these phrases contributed to moments like the one in the opening vignette of this chapter, when to my confusion a hearing person seemed to suddenly recall a deaf person.[8]

Similarly, when Sagar and I first tried to find Sarawata's house, we ended up at the wrong home, down the hillside from her actual house. We entered into conversation with an older hearing woman as she fed her cow. After ascertaining that neither Sarawata nor any other deaf person lived there, I solicited the old woman's help by asking about a married couple whose *kān nasunne* 'ears don't hear' or who *boldaina* 'don't speak.' After insisting that no one like that lived nearby, she then remembered that in fact there was a *lāṭolāṭi* couple (here, *lāṭo* is pluralized and given gender markings that indicate male and female). If I had asked for a *lāṭolāṭi* couple, would she have remembered them immediately? Interestingly, earlier I had asked a different hearing woman for directions using the phrase *kān nasunne* '[people with] not-hearing ears.'[9] Either she mistakenly thought Sarawata lived in the older woman's home, or, more likely, I followed her directions incorrectly. Either way, her response indicated that she had understood my question and connected it with Sarawata and her husband—although as the previous section showed, Sarawata could hear to some degree and as this section shows, her husband may also have been able to, again demonstrating that (not) hearing, as much as being deaf, is a social category.

In the case of the family described in the opening vignette, we had been talking about deaf people for some time, yet they "forgot" about a man who was right there when we asked if they knew other deaf people. I wonder if they were thinking about the man not in terms of him being deaf but in terms of the more immediately salient feature of their relationship: he was a client, there to get a tool fixed. Or perhaps their own granddaughter was someone they would consider "more deaf" and this difference contributed to the grandparents' "forgetting." In short, beyond a general understanding that recalling and naming persons on the basis of particular characteristics when asked to do so is a communicative task that does not necessarily "translate" across settings, I do not have a pithy analysis as to why such "forgetting" situations occurred. Yet it seems important to mention as part of a description of how hearing people thought and talked about their deaf neighbors, friends, and family members. It also turned out that Sagar and the young deaf girl's uncle had met before, and that at the initial meeting, the uncle hadn't mentioned his niece. Upon meeting the uncle again, Sagar was surprised that he hadn't mentioned his own niece was deaf. For Sagar, knowing that someone has a deaf relative is (almost) always socially relevant. For the uncle, meeting Sagar may or may not have brought to mind his niece; if it did, sharing this information apparently did not feel necessary the way that knowing that information felt necessary to Sagar.

As discussed in chapter 1, hearing villagers frequently remarked on Sagar's apparent lack of fit with their image of someone deaf, and certainly their image of someone *lāṭo*. Hearing people did not, however, regard local deaf persons as an entirely homogenous group. When differentiating among deaf people, hearing people did so in terms of either a perceived quality of mind and action that might be glossed as intelligence or competence, or a perceived capacity to use and understand speech. The people with whom I talked did not always link these qualities, although as Graif (2018) has shown, hearing people often do equate the two, and as discussed in chapter 1, deaf NSL signers explicitly dismiss this equation. A hearing man in the tea shop where we all ate after class once made a comment that no one could ever cheat Krishna, implying that he was smart and competent—and also that his being so was worth remarking on. In this particular instance, comparison with other deaf people was left implicit, while a woman with whom Sagar and I chatted when looking for several deaf people told us directly that one person we were seeking was *bāṭi* 'smart, with-it,' while the other was not.[10] (Hearing people pronounced not-always-complimentary judgments on other hearing people as well; such evaluations were not restricted to deaf people.)

Another young hearing woman I met had known at least three deaf people for her entire life, a man and a woman who came to class and a woman who did not. During our conversation this young woman noted differences between deaf people like the woman who came to class, Surya Kumari Limbu, whom she described as knowing what work she had to do and doing it well and conversing with people when they meet on the road, and people like the woman who did not participate in class, whom she said would cry when told to do something.[11] I often struggled to communicate with Surya Kumari, an important reminder that communication is always relational and context-specific. The young hearing woman also said that, unlike other deaf people, Surya Kumari almost never used her voice. This makes clear that she at least was not equating the use of speech with intelligence or competence, although some people nevertheless framed it as valuable, important, or at least worthy of comment. One deaf man's relative, for example, told me on several occasions that he could use his voice for certain words, such as *buā* 'father.' And a young woman with two deaf relatives commented on the fact that one of them was more able than the other to hear and produce words that others could understand.[12]

Despite such (perceived) differences, hearing people also classified deaf people as similar. Once, at Padma Puri's request, I spent some time talking with his mother about why it was worth his while to attend the NSL class. I suggested that he might enjoy meeting other people like himself. She replied that he already knew such people, including an elderly person down the hill from them in Bodhe, and a woman named Sarita Nepali in the other direction back toward Maunabudhuk.[13] I did not meet the elderly person in Bodhe, but Sarita was a close interlocutor, and someone whom I too would consider to be like Padma. Perhaps because our categories aligned seamlessly, Padma's mother and I did not discuss what constituted Sarita and Padma as similar from our perspectives: their perceived audiological configuration, how they communicated with their hands, how other people communicated with them using their hands, and/or something else.

Another indication that hearing people broadly perceive deaf people as similar is the fact that in Maunabudhuk and Bodhe, there were three married deaf couples currently living together, a fourth deaf couple who were separated at the time—she had moved elsewhere—but have since reunited, and one deaf woman whose late husband was deaf. Only two deaf people I knew or knew of were married to hearing people at the time of my research. While below I argue that Maunabudhuk and Bodhe are distinct from what are known as shared signing communities, the literature on such places constitutes an important source of information about deaf people's experiences in contexts other than primarily urban, institutionally-scaffolded deaf communities such as Nepal's own deaf society. In this literature, marriage—whether or not deaf people get married, and if so, to whom—is often mentioned in relation to deaf people's level of "integration" into their community, as Kusters (2010) reports. She argues, however, that the simple fact of marriage says very little; it is important to know *why* certain marriages do or do not take place. In Adamorobe, Ghana, for example, deaf-deaf marriages have been illegal since 1975 in an effort to prevent the birth of more deaf children (Kusters 2012a:348). While this ban indicates a negative evaluation of deafness, Kusters (2012a:349) describes Adamorobe in general as a "deaf-inclusive place" where "deaf people interact naturally with hearing people through sign language." The broader point, then, is that attitudes toward deaf people, and deaf people's experiences of life in hearing-majority communities, are frequently complex and even contradictory.

In Maunabudhuk and Bodhe deaf persons both "interact naturally with hearing people through sign" as they do in Adamorobe (Kusters 2012:349a) *and* struggle to do so. Here, though, deaf-deaf marriages are considered appropriate. Indeed, when an older deaf man showed up in Maunabudhuk for several days, someone jokingly suggested that he and Jyoti Limbu, a deaf woman of similar age, should get married.[14] Although I did not investigate the reasons behind deaf-deaf marriages, in this place where both love marriages and arranged marriages are common, I got the sense that families who arranged marriages for their deaf adult children with other deaf people did so on the assumption that the parents of a hearing person would not consent to a match with a deaf person, whereas the parents of a deaf person would be open to such a pairing. Such match-making implies that hearing people categorize deaf people as different from hearing people and as similar to each other.

In mid-October 2010, Sagar, Krishna, Krishna's hearing twin brother Prakash (who lived nearby), and I were signing together, and I asked why Krishna wasn't married, since Prakash was. (Although I had only met Prakash once or twice, I know that he understood my signing because he translated it into Nepali for another hearing person nearby.) Prakash replied: "*Boli na āune* 'he doesn't speak.'" Interestingly, on a different occasion, Krishna's older brother Samman said that Krishna wasn't married because they didn't have enough money.[15] Taking both statements into account, along with the fact that Krishna's living brothers were all hearing and married, it seems that being deaf and not wealthy meant Krishna had two matrimonial strikes against him. In a return visit I remember Samman telling me that he had made inquiries about a potential match for Krishna but had decided that the woman would not be a good worker, a deal-breaker in a family where—from my perspective—everyone works hard and shares labor.

Closer consideration of one of Maunabudhuk's deaf couples reveals further nuances to my descriptions of how deaf and hearing residents think of deaf people as both similar and different. Sarawata Limbu, a regular participant in NSL class, became my closest deaf interlocutor in the village. Talkative and sociable, both in class and at home, she played a key role in managing her family's three-generation household and farm. Her sister-in-law told me that Sarawata speaks and understands Limbu, and also uses her hands, and that the family communicates with her using speech and their hands (*hātle chalchha* 'doing with hands'), implying that for them to use speech alone would be insufficient.[16] My own observations and interactions with Sarawata support this characterization—although, not speaking Limbu, my ability to communicate in speech with her was obviously very limited.

Sarawata's husband, Sal Bahadur Limbu, came to class only once. When Sagar and I visited their home, we occasionally ran into him on the path there or while hanging out. He was always very shy, sometimes declining to communicate at all, although Sagar told me that he was slightly more outgoing when they were alone. I also did not have a clear sense to what degree he understood when people spoke or signed to him, but much more important, it seemed that his family did not either. As I wrote in my fieldnotes:

> His mom told a long story, which I didn't fully understand, about him being sick as a young child and having several operations on his throat, which was hugely swollen, and being taken to different wards [i.e., areas of the village] and to Biratnagar [a large city in the Tarai with better medical facilities], and I asked at some point, "So that's why he can't hear?" and she replied, "No, that's why he can't talk." And it turns out he can hear. Maybe. Sagar asked, "So he understands what people say when they talk?" And she said she didn't really know what he understands or doesn't understand but he dances when there's music (like at feasts and such) and he talks with his hands.[17]

Later in the summer, I asked Sal Bahadur's oldest younger sister "if he can hear—she said if you speak loudly, and that one ear hears and the other doesn't, but he doesn't speak, and she said he does use his hands to speak. But later I was talking with their mother, and I commented that he doesn't talk very much (meaning, communicate), and she said that was true, and he doesn't even talk very much with his hands—he'll look at her to tell her he's hungry, or make an eating gesture, but not a lot past that."[18]

The example of Sarawata and her husband shows that for hearing people, as for (some) deaf people, the production and reception of speech does not make someone not-deaf, nor necessarily does having (some) hearing. What mattered most to Sal Bahadur's family was that he, like Sarawata, uses his hands to communicate. Yet, returning to deaf people's own perspectives, Sarawata did not see them as a good match—not because he was more or less deaf than she but because he was so much less communicative. It often seemed to me that she wished for a partner with whom she could talk as volubly and easily as she did with the other deaf people in class (and with many hearing people). In other words, what presumably had made them a good match in their parents' eyes—his communicative modality and hers, the fact that the parents of a hearing person would be unlikely to consider them—did not, in her eyes or heart, make them compatible as life partners.

Some hearing villagers seemed to consider deaf people not only different from hearing people, and less likely to be accepted by them as marriage partners, but also as potentially more vulnerable to the vicissitudes of life. In late July 2010, Jyoti Limbu hurt her arm quite badly, and I went to her home to visit her and bring her tea. An older hearing neighbor from down the hill had also come to visit, and she asked why God lets deaf people be born. "[She said,] 'They feel thirst, they feel hunger, but unlike us, they cannot speak. *Na janmos* ['may they not be born'].' She painted a vivid portrait of human life as one of suffering, which is relieved by the ability to speak; either that or of human life as a series of needs which are satiated through the ability to speak (and thus get what one needs)."[19] The parents of several deaf people also expressed worries about what would happen to their adult children after they, the parents, died. Padma's mother expressed this worry in terms of love: "You have to love your disabled children the most, who else will love them, especially when we old folks die?"[20]

DEAF DEMOGRAPHY

Along with deaf and hearing people's conversations, an important source of information pertaining to the categorization of deaf people comes from government-generated lists. Scholars of South Asia and beyond have analyzed the epistemological, political, and practical complications of enumerative and classificatory projects in far more depth than is possible here (e.g., Pigg 1992; Dahal 2003; Dirks 2001). While recognizing these complications, thinking with numbers can still be productive, especially for comparisons across places and especially when there is a tradition of using such numbers for comparisons, as with scholarship on signing and deaf sociality beyond national urban settings.

In Maunabudhuk, Sagar shared with me two lists that the village had compiled as part of the process of hosting an NDFN-sponsored NSL class. The lists contained the names of twenty-five people from Maunabudhuk and nineteen from Bodhe, each person labeled *bahirā* 'deaf' or *susta shrawan* 'hard of hearing.' (I do not know if the village or NDFN initiated this distinction; I combine them into a single category.) The lists seemed fairly comprehensive if imperfect. They left off some deaf people (for example, the husband of Lalita, herself a regular class participant) and included several hearing people (for example, a young man with a cleft palate, which is perhaps significant in the linking of non-normative speech with the category *deaf*). In addition, a few people who were listed had very slight hearing disabilities but communicated easily in speech and did not seem to consider themselves, or be considered by others, deaf, *lāṭo*, or *apāṅga* 'disabled.' (One of these people nevertheless came to class on a few occasions because of its literacy training opportunities.) Toward the end of our stay in Maunabudhuk, Sagar and I revised the list for Maunabudhuk based on our experiences. While the original list had twenty-five people, our revised list had twenty-seven people, twenty-three of whom were on the original list. (We did not revise the Bodhe list because our knowledge of Bodhe was much less extensive.)

I also examined the 2011 census (Government of Nepal 2012), which lists twenty-two deaf/hard of hearing people (grouped as a single category) and three deafblind people in Maunabudhuk, with forty-two deaf/hard of hearing people and six deafblind people in Bodhe. (There is also a category of multiply disabled people that may or may not include deaf people.) While the numbers from Maunabudhuk's own list (which I have no reason to believe would have excluded deafblind people) and the 2011 census are identical, Bodhe has 2.5 times as many deaf people according to the census versus the NSL class list.

What to make of the striking discrepancy between the census, which counts forty-eight deaf people in Bodhe, and the class list, which counts nineteen? As the previous discussion has shown, this difference may be attributable to issues of ontology or epistemology ("Who is deaf?" and "What does *deaf* mean?") as well as methodology (what happens when you ask, "Do you know anyone deaf around here?"). My understanding is that a person from Maunabudhuk compiled the lists for both Maunabudhuk and Bodhe; he may not have had as much knowledge about whom, and where, to ask about deaf people in Bodhe, and asking does not necessarily (immediately) yield answers. Acknowledging the uncertainty of numbers (Jennifer Johnson-Hanks, pers. comm.), I used the different available figures to calculate a range of percentages representing deaf people as a proportion of the total populations of Maunabudhuk and Bodhe. Detailed further in appendix 1, the lowest calculated percentage for Maunabudhuk is 0.8 percent and for Bodhe is 0.6 percent, while the highest are 1.1 percent and 1.6 percent, respectively.

These percentages overlap with the low end of the range of percentages of deaf people within a total population that scholars have reported for what are often referred to as shared signing communities. Shared signing communities are generally represented as places where a sign language has emerged and become widely used by both deaf and hearing people, due to a relatively high proportion of deaf people over multiple generations, generally between 1 percent and 3 percent, often attributed to genetic causes. At particular times and places, researchers have reported a much higher percentage of deaf residents. For example, 25 percent of the population was deaf in Chilmark, on Martha's Vineyard, in the United States, at various points from the 1700s to the mid-1900s, and 11 percent of Adamorobe, Ghana, was deaf in 1961 (Kusters 2010:1, 2012a:347). However, scholars report "close to 0.6%" in Ban Khor, Thailand (Nonaka 2012); 0.75 percent in Alipur, India (Panda 2012); 1.1 percent in Adamorobe, Ghana, in 2012 (Kusters 2012a); 2.2 percent in Bengkala, Indonesia (de Vos 2012); 2.4 percent in Chican, Mexico (Delgado 2012); and 2.5–3 percent in Al-Sayyid, Israel (Kisch 2012a, 2012b). If I use the higher figures calculated for Maunabudhuk and Bodhe (1.1 percent and 1.6 percent), these are squarely within this range; if I use the lower figures (0.8 percent and 0.6 percent), they at the lower end but still within the range.

Yet I argue that Maunabudhuk and Bodhe do not constitute a shared sign community, nor does natural sign communication seem to function like a shared sign language, at least as they are classically described. Generally, the signed conversations I observed and took part in there were more tenuous than what has been documented in places like Adamorobe, Al-Sayyid, and Ban Khor. I suggest that one key reason is differences in social, spatial, and temporal densities, which can be obscured by raw numbers and even percentages. As Panda (2012:355) writes about Alipur, "deafness occurs throughout the village, but is more strongly represented in particular families, some of which have had deaf members for several continuous generations." Moreover, a map of Alipur shows a significantly higher number of deaf people in the northwest quadrant than elsewhere, and Panda (2012) reports that deafness and signing go back at least six generations. In Ban Khor, of sixteen total deaf persons, fifteen had been born in the village, and eleven of them lived in one of three subvillages (Nonaka 2009:216). The other five deaf people lived in another subvillage, and in both subvillages deaf people lived very close to one another. All but four deaf people could trace their lineages within a single extended family, and with the exception of those four, deaf people in Ban Khor at the time of Nonaka's research all had deaf siblings, a deaf parent, and/or a deaf aunt or uncle (parent's sibling) (2009:218–219). Similarly, in Al-Sayyid many deaf people have a number of deaf siblings as well as deaf relatives among extended family (Kisch 2012b:94–95). There are deaf members of each of the five major lineages in the community, and people live in "several dense clusters of multiple compounds, as well as slightly more dispersed compounds" (Kisch 2012a:366). Research on Chican, Mexico (Delgado 2012), Adamorobe, Ghana (Kusters 2012a), and Bengkala, Indonesia (de Vos 2012) also indicate that in each of these places, deaf people share family connections, live close enough that they have very frequent contact with each other, or both.

In some such settings, people cannot recall a time when there weren't both deaf and hearing residents. In Adamorobe deaf people—and presumably Adamorobe Sign Language—have been part of village life "since time immemorial" (Kusters 2014:150, quoting a hearing villager). In other places people can collectively recall when deaf children were born. In Al-Sayyid a group of deaf siblings was born between 1924 and 1940 (Kisch 2012b:91). Fewer than a hundred years later, there are a large number of deaf villagers, and "all deaf and many hearing Al-Sayyid infants are exposed to signing from birth, within the family environment, with additional (deaf or hearing) adult models in the community" (Kisch 2012a:365). In such settings communicative practices that emerge with the first generation of signers develop quickly and get transmitted through and across generations (e.g., Nonaka 2007; Sandler 2012).

In the parts of Maunabudhuk and Bodhe where I have spent time, some deaf people have deaf relatives, but there are no deaf lineages of the sort described for shared signing communities. I know three deaf people with deaf siblings. It was also reported on the village list that one deaf woman's mother was deaf; I was not able to meet her, and I did not get a clear sense from talking to other people as to how accurate this classification was. Unlike in shared signing communities, though, the majority of deaf people in Maunabudhuk and Bodhe with whom I am familiar do not have deaf relatives to whom they are related by birth or adoption, as opposed to marriage. Critically, I did not meet, nor was I told about, any kinship group with three or more deaf signers across generations, although I spent time with two sisters-in-law whose late brother and husband, respectively, was deaf. I never encountered lineages of deaf people with deaf parents, aunts and uncles, cousins, and grandparents. Moreover, in Maunabudhuk and Bodhe, four of my primary interlocutors had grown up elsewhere and married into the village. Maunabudhuk and Bodhe are multiethnic and multicaste, and there are deaf members of each of the area's major *jāt* 'caste/ethnic' groups, between which there is almost no intermarriage. In contrast, many of the above communities are endogamous; indeed, endogamy has been proposed as one of the defining characteristics of places where shared sign languages emerge (Kusters 2010).

Twelve out of twenty-two people whose homes I visited were the only deaf person in the household (Green 2014c:82). Beyond the household most deaf people in Maunabudhuk and Bodhe live close to several other deaf people, although "close" is a relative term. Many had previously met and some were in regular contact with other deaf people prior to the NSL class. By no means did they all know each other, however, nor are there geographic clusters within which deaf people tend to live. In northwest Maunabudhuk and southeast Bodhe, where I spent time and was able to map people's residences, deaf people's homes were spread quite evenly across the area (Green 2014c:82–83). These patterns of kin-based and other social relationships, both spatial and temporal, distinguish Maunabudhuk and Bodhe from shared signing communities as well as from instances where "family home-sign" (Haviland 2013) and "family sign languages" (Hou 2016) have emerged.

The relationships among deaf people and between deaf and hearing people, as well as the degree to which natural sign is shared across signers in Maunabudhuk and Bodhe, also contrast with the classic understanding of home sign. In the usual model signers are the first and usually the only signer in their social network; home sign in turn is defined as arising from a deaf signer and particular to that person (e.g., Goldin-Meadow and Mylander 1983; Goldin-Meadow 2003; Coppola, Spaepen, and Goldin-Meadow 2013).[21] In Maunabudhuk and Bodhe deaf signers' repertoires are more than incidentally conventional and mutually intelligible. I discuss, and complicate, the relationship of conventionality to mutual intelligibility in chapter 3, but as a brief example, take the following. On June 1, I showed Krishna and his family, including his hearing brother Samman, a few clips of video that I had recently filmed in class and at Sarawata's house: "I translated some of what Sagar was saying in the first couple films, especially when he was teasing people. Samman really enjoyed that, and would laugh when he could see that someone else was teasing Sagar. [When he saw the film from Sarawata's house,] he translated what the neighbor . . . said to Sarawata's husband: she was teasing him that Sagar might steal his wife."[22]

Sarawata's neighbor and Samman live on opposite sides of the village and come from different *jāt* 'caste/ethnic' and language backgrounds. According to their own reports, prior to the NSL class, Sarawata and Krishna had never met (though Sarawata had seen Krishna), precluding the possibility that they had co-created or merged linguistic repertoires and then passed those repertoires back to their families. The fact that Krishna's hearing brother was nevertheless able to understand and translate what Sarawata's hearing neighbor had signed suggests that some conventions in local natural sign are widely shared among both deaf and hearing people. Relatedly, as a learner, I did not have to acquire individualized repertoires for each deaf person with whom I spent time in Maunabudhuk and Bodhe, even if I came to recognize particular signs or pragmatic patterns as specific to individuals. And Sagar could easily communicate with both deaf and hearing people—a testament, to be sure, to his communicative skills and also evidence of some conventionality.

Given that not all deaf people in the area knew each other or spent time together, this conventionality in turn suggests that even in the absence of spatial and familial clusters of signers, people transmit signs across time and space (Nyst, Sylla, and Magassouba [2012] suggest something similar). Sagar, Prajwal, and Furba's descriptions in chapter 1 of deaf children learning natural signs from hearing people support this claim. In fact, the existence of both differences and similarities in signs across different Nepali setting are evidence of multiple, variously scaled semiotic traditions. The sign GIRL/WOMAN, for example, is the same in Maunabudhuk and Kathmandu but different in Atharasaya, the village directly across the valley on Maunabudhuk's eastern side. The negating sign, however, is in use not only across Nepal but also India and according to Adam Schembri (pers. comm.) in other parts of Asia as well.

Discussion of transmission implicates the temporal axis in the literature on signing classifications. Meir et al. (2010) propose the category of emerging sign languages, contrasting with established sign languages. Emerging sign languages cut across sociospatial axes, including, for example, Al-Sayyid Bedouin Sign Language, a shared sign language (Meir et al. use the term "village sign language"), and Israeli Sign Language, which they call a "deaf community sign language." What these languages share is a relatively recent and rapid emergence, characterized by significant linguistic change, over a few generations or cohorts of signers. In the case of Israeli Sign Language this emergence is tied to the founding of deaf schools and other institutions, while in the case of Al-Sayyid it is tied to increasing numbers of deaf people born into the village (Meir et al. 2010). As discussed in chapter 1, NSL has emerged recently and rapidly, at least in part from natural sign, and thus could be classified as an emerging sign language (as well as a deaf community sign language).[23]

In Maunabudhuk and Bodhe, where no one shared with me a collective memory of a time prior to which deaf people were not present in the region, there is no evidence that natural sign is new, young, or quickly changing. This lack of a pre-deaf epoch motivates my choice not to use a framework that positions hearing people's co-speech gestures as the material from which deaf people develop signs, despite the fact that hearing speakers in Nepal use a rich gestural repertoire that overlaps with natural sign.[24] Without evidence I do not want to assume that this repertoire began by belonging only to hearing people. It is also hard to predict if and how natural sign might change in the future. In Maunabudhuk and Bodhe there are not families or neighborhoods in which there are large, and growing, numbers of deaf people, so it does not seem likely that natural sign will become a conventional signed language in this region, although as more and more children attend deaf schools, the way they use natural sign after learning NSL could certainly affect the broader usage of natural sign in their home communities, including Maunabudhuk and Bodhe. Here it is worth noting that in Kathmandu, natural sign continues to exist and be used both by non-NSL signers and by NSL signers, including young people.[25]

It is for these reasons that I use the term *emergent* to describe natural sign, both generally in Nepal and specifically in Maunabudhuk and Bodhe. *Emergent* in contrast to *emerging* emphasizes that natural sign is not necessarily new and does not have a predictable trajectory. *Emergent* in contrast to *conventional* highlights that signers and addressees have to do a great deal of sense-making work (although conventional language practices are also emergent, and emergent language practices involve conventionality, as discussed in chapter 3).[26] I also want to stress that Maunabudhuk and Bodhe are not considered unusual places in Nepal; they are not referred to by residents as having particularly high numbers of deaf people, nor did anyone at the NDFN imply that they were when we discussed the three or four places hosting NSL classes in 2010. Sagar himself had previously taught in two other locales in the same district. Indeed, the fact that NSL outreach classes have been ongoing for several decades implies that many places in Nepal are home to a "high" number of deaf people.[27]

Annelies Kusters (pers. comm.) suggests that the situation I have described in Maunabudhuk and Bodhe may in fact characterize the most common kind of communicative setting for deaf people in the world. Zeshan (2011:228–229) makes a similar argument—namely that situations in which "a number of deaf individuals . . . are in sporadic, unsystematic contact with each other" are, "far from being something extraordinary, . . . actually a common occurrence." She ascribes the resulting communicative practices, which she calls "communal homesign," only to deaf people's contact with other deaf people, whereas natural sign is clearly a product of interaction both among deaf people and between deaf and hearing people.

My point is not that deaf people are not critical in the development of signing practices, but that the presence of deaf people in the social field and of signed forms in the linguistic field are not exceptional. Here I am in conversation with disability studies and disability justice scholars and activists (e.g., Ginsburg and Rapp 2017; Piepzna-Samarasinha 2022) who sharply critique mainstream, and mainstream social scientists', understanding of disability as anomalous rather than as regular, even common: experienced, to be sure, in particular ways in particular times and places but never absent. In the same vein, sustained attention to deaf experiences shows that while particular places may not have deaf residents for some period of time, in most times and places the social world has never just been hearing. Space-time has never not been deaf.

A BRIEF, FURTHER INDULGENCE IN TERMINOLOGIES AND TAXONOMIES

My goals in this chapter have been multiple: to think carefully about the categories, classifications, and taxonomies present both in the ethnographic and scholarly fields with which I am most engaged; and to open up the logics of the latter to those of the former. Moreover, *natural sign* and *local sign*, the two terms that I have borrowed or adapted from my interlocutors in Nepal and sought to put into conversation with extant scholarly ones, both demand further specificity and offer purchase into each other.

Using the word *local* is one of the ways—the only one involving English—that Nepali speakers in Maunabudhuk referred to the signing practices in use among themselves and their deaf relatives and neighbors. In Nepal the designation *local* conveys both a sense of ownership and belonging *and* a sense of fraught comparison to elsewhere. To give a concrete example, there are two types of *ambā* 'guava' in Maunabudhuk. The fruits of one type are small and tasty whether hard or fully ripened; these are known as *local* guavas. So-called *bikāsit* 'developed' guavas, meanwhile, are larger, sweeter, and pink inside (and no doubt fetch more per kilo) but are only edible when ripe. According to Fortier (2009), the term *local* also relates closely to the Nepali *prākriti* 'nature, natural.' She writes: "Local places . . . are thought of as *prākriti* . . . or a local dialect is called *Prākrit*, the natural language of the local people" (Fortier 2009:60). In contrast to the quality of being *sanskriti* (cultural), that which is *prākriti* "contains an *emergent* quality that is *contingent on local circumstances*" (Fortier 2009:60–61, emphases added).[28] The Nepali, and perhaps broader South Asian, understandings of both *local* and *natural* emphasize particularity and contingency. As I understand them, both the terms *local* and *natural* demand empirical specificity. Hence I use them both as categories and also as placeholders that direct further examination.

CONCLUSION

This chapter has literally and figuratively located deaf users of natural sign in Maunabudhuk and Bodhe in relation to each other and to existing classificatory frameworks of deaf people and signing practices. I explored deaf and hearing residents' perspectives on the category *deaf*, particularly in relation to sensory and communicative configurations. In concert with Kusters's (2010) critical point that researchers should pay attention to the subjective experiences of deaf persons beyond large signing communities, I suggested that doing so involves asking questions such as: "What does deaf mean?" "Who is deaf?" "How might I as a researcher know who is deaf?" Moreover, even seemingly straightforward yes-or-no questions like "Can you hear?" are no less socially specific than questions like "What are deaf people's experiences?"

Seeking both to be in conversation with the rich and important literature on deaf socialities and communication and to push against the flattening effects of taxonomies, I showed how natural sign differs from extant scholarly categories in terms of the associated spatial, familial, and temporal relationships among signers. This demographically-oriented account further explains and elaborates on local natural sign's paradoxical possibilities and precarities. In Maunabudhuk and Bodhe there are not dense clusters of deaf relatives and neighbors, among whom (and among whose hearing relatives and neighbors), natural sign would be a primary language; natural sign is not the communicative medium of a tightly connected group of people with a consistent need and desire to sign. Usage patterns, however, suggest that some natural sign forms are transmitted across time and widely available for use. Given these circumstances, it is unsurprising that natural sign communication is often easy and often difficult.

The demand for specificity invoked at the end of this chapter is answered in chapter 3 in two ways: (1) by describing and analyzing particular examples of signs and utterances from Maunabudhuk and Bodhe, and (2) by theorizing the affordances and limits of natural sign through a consideration of the relationship between linguistic and other bodily and social conventions or habits. This theorization arises specifically from my work with natural sign in Maunabudhuk and Bodhe, while providing a general framework that can be used to analyze other emergent language practices. Chapter 3 also further elaborates on natural sign's contradictions: it involves conventions, but it is not conventional language; it is readily available, but it requires work; it is known in the body, but it can be easily dismissed as unknowable, as explored in chapters 4 and 5.

Making Sense

3

Semiotics

In late September 2010, as we waited at the tea shop across the street from the village hall for class to begin, Padma Puri was signing to me about farming. I wrote in my fieldnotes later that I was pretty sure I understood when he made reference to the process of making and weeding terraces. As for what crop he was telling me about, however, I struggled: I "couldn't figure it out—[I] kept getting stuck on rice vs millet," two of the major terraced crops in the area, and ones I had watched people plant or participated in planting myself. When Padma continued the conversation with Sagar Karki in the classroom, Sagar immediately understood that Padma was talking about lentils. I expressed frustration with not having been able to understand that, or the ensuing conversation about planting methods. Sagar asked me, "Well, do you habitually plant lentils?" I wrote in my fieldnotes: "Good point, practically and theoretically."[1]

Here I use Sagar's comment as an entry into taking seriously the relationship between the capacity to produce and interpret signs and the experience of living in a particular world. As part of this book's commitment to emancipatory pragmatics (Hanks, Ide, and Katagiri 2009) and to centering deaf epistemologies (Kusters, De Meulder, and O'Brien 2017), I treat his question as arising from embodied and objectifiable knowledge of communicating in natural sign, and not as a misapprehension or mistake. I follow his insight, and natural sign's practical and theoretical demands, by both holding apart and dissolving the line between linguistic and nonlinguistic conventions, including those that might be described as bodily movements (signing, other actions), social knowledge, pragmatic tendencies, and habit. I explore the interrelated practical and theoretical implications of (thinking about) making and understanding reference being at least partially dependent on and motivated by nonlinguistic modes of being in and knowing a world—such as familiarity with planting lentils. Focusing on particular examples will hopefully give readers a sense of the materiality of natural sign. Through these examples I develop a semiotic framework for thinking about why "knowing" natural sign is neither sufficient nor exactly necessary for communicating in it.

This framework draws on and further theorizes three key concepts: *conventionality, immanence,* and *emergence.* Each of these concepts addresses how a sign means something to someone or, in the language of semiotician Charles Peirce (1955:99), "stands to somebody for something in some respect or capacity." *Conventionality* describes the property of a sign, or a combination of signs, being repeatable and/or shared. Another way of saying this is that conventionality is twofold: how stable signs are within a signer's repertoire and how shared signs are across signers' repertoires.[2] Conventional signs are ones that people "know" the way you, as a reader, and I, as a writer, know the words in this sentence and how they relate to one another syntactically. Conventional signs mean something because they're familiar as signs.

Immanence refers to a nonarbitrary relational quality among a sign's form, the sociomaterial world, and the sign's referent. In technical terms immanence highlights how signs may be interpreted—whether in conversation or in the context of a scholarly account—iconically (through resemblance or similarity) or indexically (through proximity or association).[3] Put another way, immanent signs materialize and exhibit a not-just-linguistic connection or series of connections between the bodily articulation of a sign and what it stands for. The consequence of this immanence is that such signs are potentially make-able and interpretable in context without prior linguistic conventionality for signer and/or addressee. It is worth noting that particular natural signs might be both conventional and immanent, or conventional to one person and immanent to another. And, crucially, both conventionality and immanence offer affordances or possibilities for people to understand what has been signed, but also limitations.

Emergence refers to the way that signs in combination take on meaning in relation to each other. In interpreting signers' utterances, addressees can draw on some conventional grammatical and pragmatic patterns, but there is also a need for significant inferential work or guesswork. Immanence gets at what is already there *in potentia* but must be brought into being through articulation. Emergence gets at what further elaborative work must be done with what has been provided, with what is happening in real time. Imagistically, I think of immanence as grounded, emergence as growing. In natural sign, making and making sense of utterances requires both.

Both immanence and emergence point to how meaning-making in natural sign involves conventions of various sorts. In the case of immanence, the conventions are twofold: sociomaterial (the way another village is visible across a valley, the height of corn, the motion of a hand tenderly painting dots on a sibling's forehead) and modal (the use of pointing to direct an addressee's attention to that village, the use of an arm held in space to indicate height, the use of a hand moving up one's own forehead to stand for an action that in a different context would be performed on another's body). In the case of emergence, the conventions are twofold in a different sense: formal (the recognition that a thumb held up means THE-OLDEST—i.e., a conventional sign) and pragmatic (the recognition that a thumb held up at this moment means 'oldest daughter' but at that moment 'oldest sister').[4] Yet as I show in this chapter, immanence and emergence also demand that signers and addressees make meaning in ways that are not fully captured by the idea of conventionality. I locate the possibility of understanding at least in part in the corporeal fact that people have, and are, bodies and live in particular sociomaterial spaces with others.

A FURTHER NOTE ON METHOD AND THEORY

My insistence on the importance of bodies entails recognition of the role that my own experience has played in my efforts to characterize natural sign and its semiotics. What did I learn as a conventional sign? What could I draw on as immanent right away? What became immanent as I spent more time in Maunabudhuk? When I did, or did not, understand someone's signs, was this (lack of) understanding due to my knowledge of the signs as conventions, my sense of their immanence in the world, or both? It is also important to note that these categories were nowhere close to fully fleshed out while I was doing fieldwork, so I did not write fieldnotes using such words, making some of the analytic work of deciphering what I wrote about the processes of my own and others' understanding even more challenging.

In theorizing immanence, I am building on a long tradition of investigating the relationships between form and meaning, sign and signer, community and communication. Scholars have written about signs as decipherable to more and less socially proximate people (Kuschel 1973), as context-dependent (Washabaugh, Woodward, and DeSantis 1978), and as context-sensitive (Green 2011), as well as about the role of shared social knowledge in language structure (Padden 2011). The specific semiotic and linguistic devices through which signs are articulated and (at least potentially) understood have been framed as characterizing, constructed action, decipherability, depicted action, iconicity, image, indexicality, pantomime, transparency, and whole body classifiers among other terms (Kendon 1980b; Pizzuto and Volterra 2000; Taub 2001; Liddell 2003; Padden et al. 2013; Cormier, Smith, and Sehyr 2015; Padden et al. 2015; Green 2017; Graif 2018; Hodge, Ferrara, and Anible 2019; Hoffmann-Dilloway 2021; Caselli, LIeberman, and Pyers 2021). Throughout this book, and in this chapter in particular, I both make use of and push against many of these approaches, sometimes at the same moment.

While Hanks (1993:152) asks that linguists and linguistic anthropologists—traditionally concerned with spoken language—"see the literal core of language as already permeated by context," scholars of gesture and sign have been less able to ignore this quality of permeation.[5] Yet this scholarship has not always given enough attention to the sociomaterial complexities and entanglements of bodies, places, and semiotic processes. In conversation with a linguistic ethnography approach to deaf people's communication (Kusters and Hou 2020), I draw on Hanks's practice-based approach in hopes of reanimating, or repeopling, sign linguistics' long-standing investment in taking form seriously. I seek to emphasize that making and making sense of signs—producing immanent signs, interpreting them, elaborating on a lean utterance with relevant knowledge of events, places, or people—are social actions done by specific people in specific places.

Hanks's (1990) approach to communication as social practice recognizes that grammatical structures are patterned in systematic ways and that people use language in routine but not predetermined ways. Bringing together practice theory, in particular Pierre Bourdieu's work (e.g., 1972 [1977]), and phenomenology, especially Maurice Merleau-Ponty's (1945 [1967]) and Alfred Schutz's (1970) scholarship, Hanks situates language use in the socially habituated body of culturally situated actors and emphasizes the importance of place as itself comprised of dynamic relationships, a kind of dense accrual (similar to Massey [1994]). In communicative as in other social practices, each iteration—each word, gesture, utterance, conversation—becomes part of the schematic ground from which the next iteration arises. Goodwin (2018) similarly emphasizes the scaffolding and reuse of resources in his approach to communication as cooperative action. People encounter, embody, produce, and remake the habitual forms of practice that characterize their social worlds. This process of (re)production helps explain how language in use is conventional but creative, continuous with the past but always changing, patterned but not determined. Moreover, habit, or *habitus* to use Bourdieu's term, is implicated in communicative practice not only in the forms employed but also in the orientations and schemas people use to produce actual utterances and to understand each other. These forms, orientations, and schemas do not exist in isolation but are instead part of social and linguistic fields that are in turn mutually embedded in each other (Hanks 1990, 1996).

I turn now to a brief description of Maunabudhuk and Bodhe as sociomaterial fields. The next section further explores conventionality and immanence, while the final section addresses conventionality and emergence.

FIELDS

Located in the southeastern corner of Dhankuta district in eastern Nepal, Maunabudhuk and Bodhe lay draped across the hills, such that from many vantage points one can see nearby houses and fields, neighboring villages (figure 11), the district's eponymous headquarters, and, in the cooler, clearer months, the massive white peaks of the Himalayas. Numerous well-trod footpaths curve along the

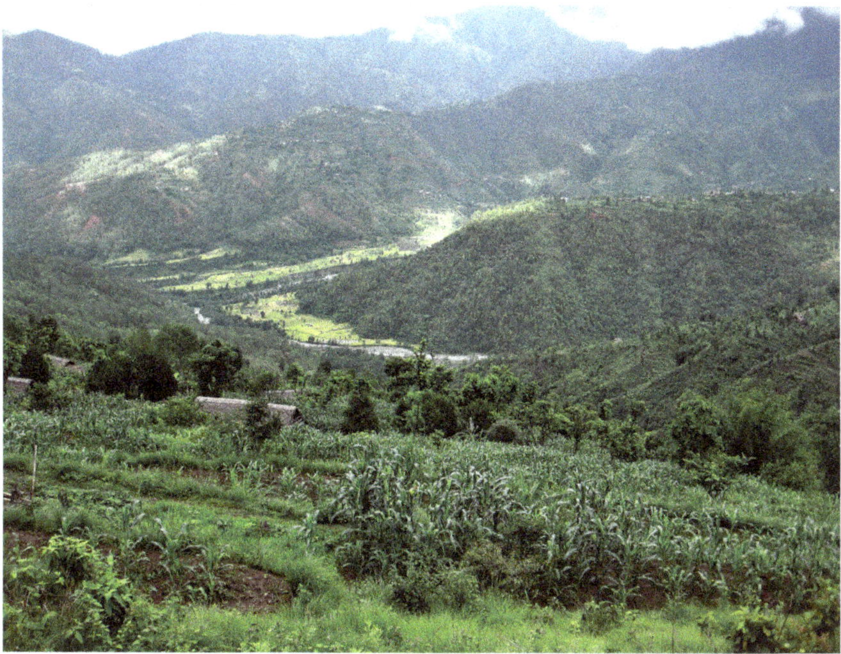

FIGURE 11. View in July 2010 on the way to Krishna's house from the bazaar: a terraced slope leads down to a bright green river valley from which a series of hills rises implacably. Photograph from the author's archives.

slopes or zigzag up and down them, connecting houses, grazing areas, fruit trees, water taps, fields, gardens, and forests. Several wide dirt roads—leveled by bulldozers—also wind through the villages. Maunabudhuk's bazaar (figure 12) is located on such a road, dusty or muddy with the changing seasons. When I lived there, the government primary school sat at the south end, while the government secondary school, the private primary school, and an open soccer field sat at the north end. In between were the village government offices and health post, along with houses and shops constructed from concrete and wood. Storefronts and boarding houses offered ready-made clothes, medicine, sewing services, umbrellas, beauty supplies, fertilizer, foodstuff, watch repair, a place to stay for the night, and assorted meals, snacks, hot tea, and alcohol.[6]

In 2010 both villages had populations of about three thousand people. In Maunabudhuk, according to its own data that was shared with me, about two-thirds of its residents were Limbu, 17 percent were Bahun or Chhetri, and 6 percent were Dalit, with Rai and other caste/ethnic groups making up the remainder of the population. In Bodhe, according to the 2011 census, 38 percent were Yakkha, Rai, or Yamphu, 25 percent were Bahun and Chhetri, 10 percent were Limbu, and 9 percent were Dalit, with Tamang and other caste/ethnic groups making up the

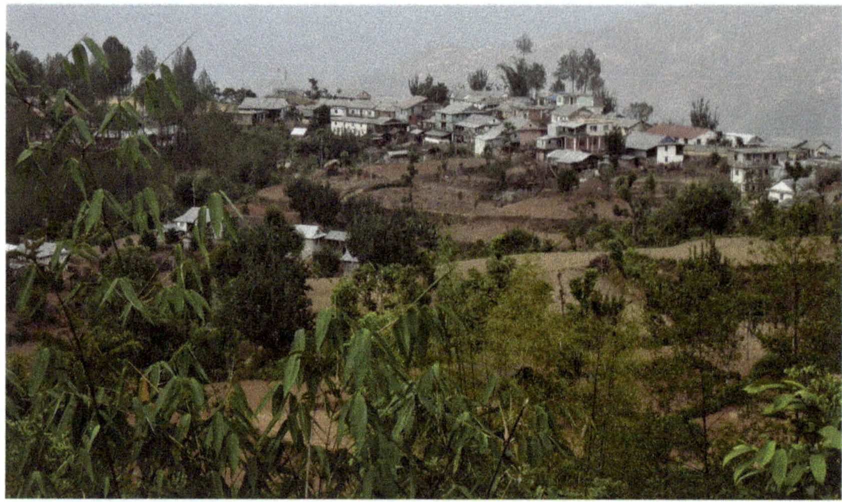

FIGURE 12. View in May 2010 on the way to Sarawata's house: the bazaar—a clustered row of white, pale teal, and brick-red buildings—contrasts with the surrounding brown fields and dark green foliage. Photograph from the author's archives.

rest. Within Nepal's ethnic/caste system, Limbus, Rais, Yamphus, and Yakkhas—all of whom are grouped together as Kiranti—are, along with Tamangs, classified as *janājāti* 'ethnic' groups. Bahuns, Chhetris, and Dalits, meanwhile, are considered to be *jāt* 'caste' groups, with Bahuns and Chhetris historically considered "high" and Dalits "low" or untouchable. In everyday parlance people use the term *jāt* for both caste and ethnic groups, and in nineteenth- and early twentieth-century legislation, ethnic groups such as Limbus and Rais were placed in a mid-level between high castes and Dalits (Hofër 2004). While *jāt*-based discrimination is illegal in Nepal, Maunabudhuk, like the rest of Nepal, continues to be shaped by locally-specific relations of hierarchy, discrimination, resistance, affiliation, and intimacy in social, economic, and political spheres (e.g., M. Cameron 1998; Caplan 2000 [1970]; Fisher 2001; Guneratne 2002; Dahal 2003; Green 2022b). The people with whom I interacted on a regular basis—both deaf and hearing—were primarily Limbu, Dalit, Chhetri, and Bahun, reflecting not only the ratio of these groups within the broader population but also their spatial distribution within the villages.

Nepali is the native language of Bahuns, Chhetris, and Dalits, while many Limbu, Rai, Yakkha, and Tamang families speak Nepali as well as Limbu, Rai, Yakkha, or Tamang (these terms may themselves encompass distinct dialects or languages). The 2011 census lists Limbu as the mother language of the entire Limbu population in Maunabudhuk, indexing the salience of mother tongue politics in Nepal but masking the massive language shift toward Nepali among younger generations. Reflecting the history of linguistic, cultural, and economic dominance by "high"-caste Nepali speakers, Nepali is the primary medium in the local government offices and schools, and in conversations between people from Nepali-speaking and other linguistic backgrounds. I did, however, hear Limbu spoken, not only in homes but in Maunabudhuk's bazaar as well. I have no doubt that other languages such as Rai are also spoken in homes and the bazaar.

Most families in Maunabudhuk, regardless of *jāt*, are primarily farmers. As I learned from observations and conversations, especially with village official Ganga Limbu, the major field crops are corn and millet, mostly used for subsistence purposes. Although many people eat rice for the two major daily meals, few families in Maunabudhuk grow rice, at least in the more elevated areas where my primary interlocutors live, as this higher-up land is not sufficiently irrigated. The two biggest cash crops are *nāspāti* 'Asian pear' and *suntalā* 'orange'; raising pigs and chickens also provides a source of extra income for some. Other livestock include goats (used and sold for meat), cows (milk), and water buffalos (meat or milk). In addition, nearly every household in Maunabudhuk relies on remittances from family members—mostly men—working abroad, especially in the Gulf States or Malaysia. Locally, people earn money working on construction sites, loading trucks, or doing other manual labor, or as teachers and healthcare providers. Some families rent or own the shops mentioned above, offering a place to stay, snacks and meals, school and farming supplies, as well as services like sewing or blacksmithing. These latter occupations are strongly but not strictly correlated with *jāt*. On Saturday mornings farmers from the surrounding area line the street near the village offices with piles of assorted fruits and vegetable; at the other end of the bazaar, near the government primary school, butchers offer chunks of fresh meat, and women sell fermented grain alcohol.

Agricultural, domestic, and other labor activities, and the built spaces in which they occur, are embedded in and productive of a dense field of sociality. As in the Nepali village described by Ahearn (2001:13), people in Maunabudhuk and Bodhe spend much of their time outside: on porches, in courtyards, at personal or communal water taps, in fields and grazing areas. Family members perform some and frequently all of their own agricultural labor: cutting grass for fodder, grazing and feeding animals, hauling water, chopping firewood, hoeing and plowing fields, weeding, harvesting, and storing crops. Relatives and neighbors may also work together in turn or hire people for labor. While products such as rice, tea, and sugar are readily available in the bazaar stores, many everyday consumption items—such as millet- and corn-based beer and hard liquor, cornmeal, *achār* 'pickles, hot sauces'—are produced at home.

When home, people nearly always keep their doors open, and someone is often outside, anyway, on the porch or in the garden. In Maunabudhuk's bazaar, the small tea shops and restaurants are open on the street side, allowing interactions between patrons and passersby. People also frequently sit in front of stores to pass time talking together, while kids run between their own and their friends' homes. In the rest of the village, fields surround some houses such that the nearest

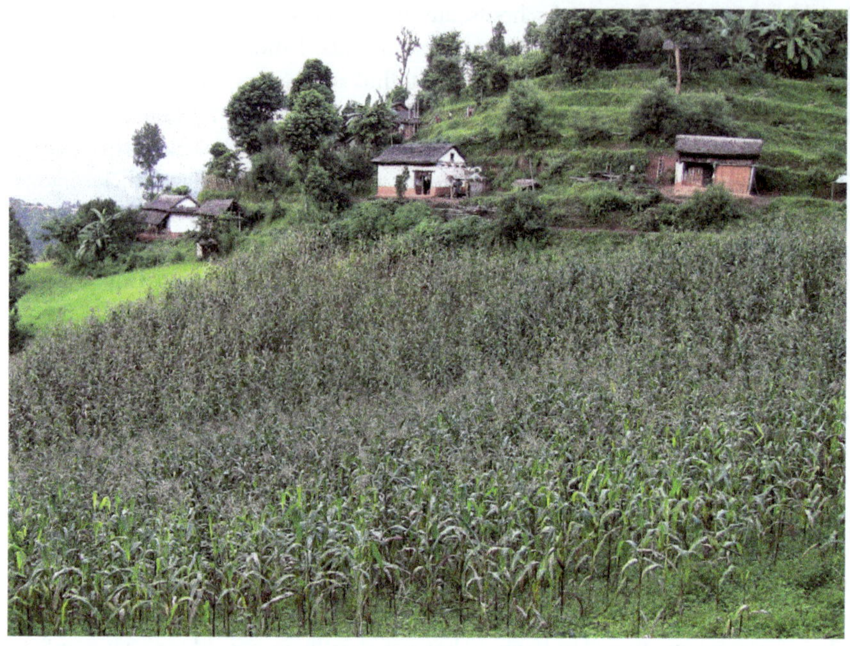

FIGURE 13. The hamlet where Sarita lived: several small, thatch-roofed homes, neatly painted with whitewash and clay, nestle between a cornfield and a terraced slope. Photograph from the author's archives.

neighbors are a few minutes' walk away, while other houses are built in clusters or hamlets (figure 13). During most of my visits to people's homes, I met not only members of the household but also other relatives and neighbors, some of whom came to see the foreign anthropologist and the "handsome" deaf Nepali, others of whom were dropping by for social and/or work-related purposes.

People travel not only within the area but also beyond it, with buses carrying people—and goods—between Maunabudhuk and the district headquarters as well as Dharan, at the edge of the plains, both a few hours' drive on winding roads. Along with buses, tractors carrying loads of construction material, an ambulance used to transport serious cases from the local health clinic to a larger hospital, and the occasional motorcycle plied Maunabudhuk's roads, but usually they served as exceptionally broad footpaths for people and livestock.

The conventional greetings people give each other along pathways reflect the salience of movement in everyday life, including noting and acknowledging others' movements. "*Kahā̃ bāṭa āunubhaeko* 'Where are you coming from?'" "*Kahā̃ jānubhaeko* 'Where are you going?'" Such questions are asked even when the answers are obvious, as when children would sing out, "*O didi, nuhāuna jānubhaeko* 'Hey older sister, are you going to bathe?'" as I walked the hundred meters from my home to the nearest water tap bearing a bucket of laundry, shampoo, and soap.

TABLE 1 The quadrants

Quadrant 1:	Quadrant 2:
More conventional, more immanent	Less conventional, more immanent
Quadrant 3:	Quadrant 4:
More conventional, less immanent	Less conventional, less immanent

CONVENTIONALITY AND IMMANENCE

There are widespread conventions in natural sign. At least some of these conventions are also immanent in the world in which signers live and communicate, and thus possibly, though not necessarily, interpretable without prior knowledge of sign forms as signs. Immanence affords signers and addressees with the ability to make and understand signs even in the absence of (knowledge of) linguistic conventions. While this point might seem to imply that conventionality and immanence are opposites, it is more helpful to think about them as gradient qualities along perpendicular axes.[7] These axes produce four quadrants: more conventional and more immanent signs, less conventional and more immanent signs, more conventional and less immanent signs, and less conventional and less immanent signs (table 1).

Conventional natural signs that are less immanent (quadrant 3) need to be known as signs. In Peircian (1955) terms, such signs are symbolic legisigns. They would not be decipherable (Kuschel 1973) from the relationship between their form and everyday nonlinguistic context (though one might be able to figure out their meaning from the broader utterance or conversation in which they get used). One example of a sign that I experienced as conventional and nonimmanent is shown in figure 14a; I gloss this sign NEG, short for 'negator,' because it is used to indicate that something is not true, not available, doesn't exist, and so forth. Another sign, figure 14b, functions as a general wh-question; I gloss it Q. The people depicted, Surya Kumari Limbu and Padma Puri, are deaf residents of Maunabudhuk and Bodhe who participated in the NSL class.[8]

Other conventional natural signs are also immanent (quadrant 1). As discussed earlier, immanence gets at the potential availability of the sociomaterial world for transformation, articulation, and rendering through bodily movement (including pointing). Affordances are a classic way of thinking about this potential, and in sign language research, affordances are often framed in relation to signing as a modality. I want to think here as well about the affordances of the world and about their convergence with the affordances of signing. The world nudges signers to reach for certain representational devices, as with the circular movement of a fist to represent grinding flour or pointing to the forehead in an upward line to represent a holiday where colored dots are applied to the forehead, discussed in the introduction. Immanence can be grounded not only in bodily routines, but also in

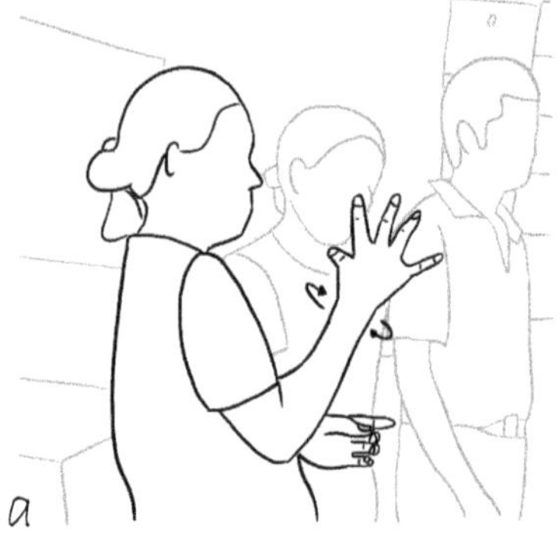
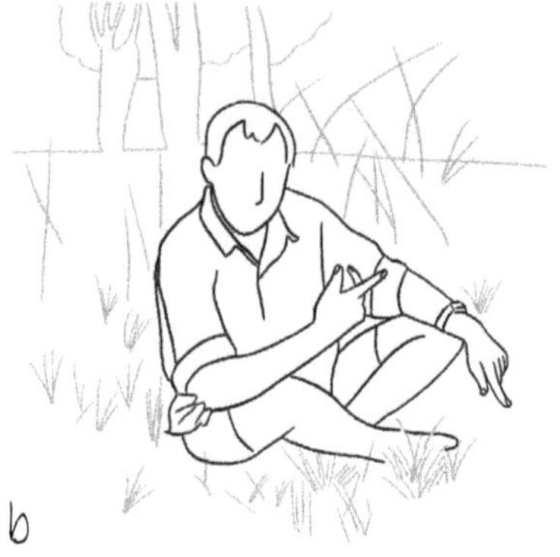

FIGURE 14. (a) Standing in the village hall with other signers, Surya Kumari Limbu signs the negating sign, her open hand held upright and rotating at the wrist. (b) Seated in a field, Padma Puri signs the general wh-question sign, one hand with thumb and forefinger extended flipping from palm down to palm up (the sign can also be made two-handed). Illustrations by Nanyi Jiang.

landscapes, in histories, in the way plants grow or animals eat, in the movement of the sun from east to west.[9]

Kendon (1980b, calling on Mandel 1977) refers to what gets drawn on in a sign's articulation as its base. This classification usefully highlights the specificity of sign by distinguishing between related-yet-distinct actions conducted for different purposes—doing a thing versus talking about it, such as making grain alcohol versus referring to it—and grounding the latter in the former. The distinction between the form and base—a distinction that sign language linguistics often collapses—makes it possible to demonstrate *how* the world shows up in signs and not only *that* it does. It reveals how sign forms are immanent in the "routine patterns of experience and interaction through which actors [encounter and] recognize objects, individuals, and events not as mere things but as instances of familiar categories" (Hanks 1990:70, citing Schutz 1970).

The way that signers actually materialize this immanence—in the directions their fingers point, the shapes they trace, the actions they pantomime—makes use of two key bodily and semiotic strategies. First, they make use of the capacity of the body to draw attention to features of the environment that are sensorially accessible to their addressees (Hanks 1990; Edwards 2015). In Peirce's terminology these are indexical signs; in Kendon's these are pointing and presenting signs. For example, someone might point at a person or grasp a necklace. Second, signers make use of the capacity of the body to enact similitude to movements, qualities, or features; these signs would be known as iconic, in Peirce's terms, and as characterizing or enacting, in Kendon's. For example, someone could hold one hand as if gripping a bundle of grass, the other making a slashing motion underneath it as if cutting fodder. Many signs (not just natural signs, and not just signs in the sense of signing practices) make use of both of these strategies simultaneously (Peirce

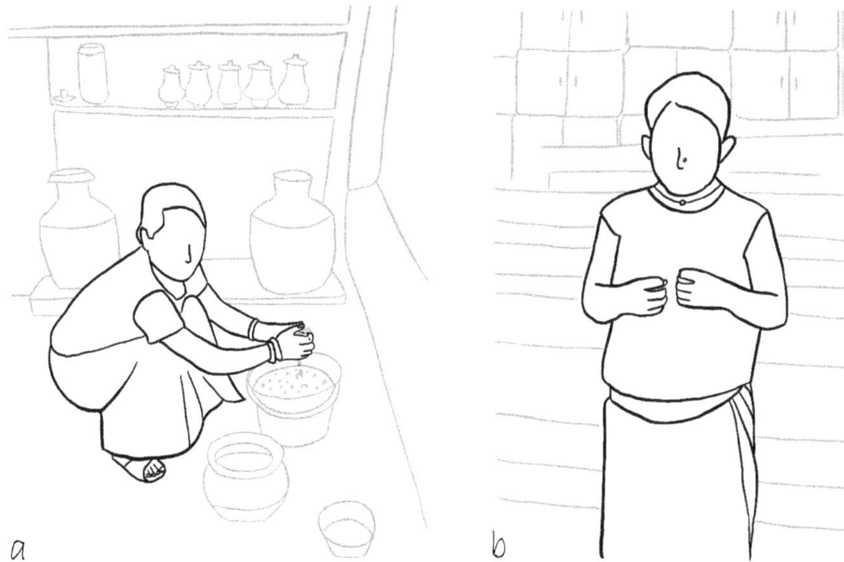

FIGURE 15. (a) Sarawata Limbu squats in her kitchen, squeezing the liquid of fermenting millet and corn from her hands back into a container. (b) Jyoti Limbu stands in the village hall, signing "GRAIN-ALCOHOL," her fingers squeezing into loose fists as the hands move toward each other. Illustrations by Nanyi Jiang.

1955). For example, placing one's hand at the height of a child could be interpreted as both iconic and indexical.

In the case of the sign GRAIN-ALCOHOL, the base is the motion that someone makes as she squeezes liquid from a handful of fermenting grains, as Sarawata Limbu is doing in figure 15a. The form of the sign reproduces that squeezing movement, as shown by Jyoti Limbu in figure 15b.[10] The sign, in other words, is immanent in the bodily process of making alcohol. Many other signs used in Maunabudhuk and Bodhe are similarly articulated with a "movement pattern . . . consist[ing] of a selection from elements of action that would be performed if the action sequence or pattern being characterized were actually being carried out" (Kendon 1980b:87).

Continuing to think with Kendon (1980b), signs have not only bases and forms but also referents. A referent has one of multiple possible relationships to its base, depending on the specific utterance (Kendon 1980b:85, 89–97). In an utterance where the referent is the alcohol itself, then the representation of the process stands for the product; in an utterance where the referent is the making of grain alcohol, the representation of the process stands for the process. Recognizing these kinds of standing-for relationships enables a precise accounting of the complex semiotics involved that moves beyond labeling signs as iconic/indexical, or even as more or less iconic/indexical.

As another example, the sign in Maunabudhuk and Bodhe for GIRL/WOMAN involves taking one hand, with fingers separated and loosely bent, and brushing it a few times through one's hair on the side of the head above the ear, or, if the signer is bald, through the space where hair would be. The relationship between the sign form (what the hands do) and the base (the actual act of combing hair) might be described as characterizing (the hand takes on the characteristics of a brush or comb) and enacting (making a brushing motion), to use Kendon's terms; or, the base could be thought of as having hair long enough to comb, in which case the relationship of form to base would be characterizing or indicating the length of hair via its combability. The base-referent relationship, as per Kendon, could be said to involve an action standing for a person (the kind of person typified as brushing hair) or a trait standing for a person (the kind of person typified as having long hair). Signers and addressees know, of course, that men and boys comb their hair too; and that men and boys may have long hair, and women and girls may have short hair. Nevertheless, the association of women and girls with longer hair and more elaborate hair care routines than their male counterparts is a social fact. In this sense, the sign, while conventional, is also immanent in the sense that it draws on bodily practices interpreted through a "cultural stock[s] of conventional typifications" (Enfield 2006:408, citing Schutz 1970; note also Hanks 1990 and Green 2022b).

The signs just analyzed—GRAIN-ALCOHOL, GIRL/WOMAN—are examples of signs that are both conventional and immanent (quadrant 1). Kendon (1980b:83) cautions that "the modes of signification" he analyzes "do not necessarily play a part in the process by which a sign serves to convey its meaning to its recipient."[11] At the same time, he argues that "there is no doubt that the potential for visual iconicity available in gesturing is widely exploited by signers. Signers will resort to a variety of devices of direct visual expression whenever they are confronted with the need to say something for which no ready-made sign exists" (Kendon 1980b:82–83). Once, for example, Jyoti Limbu, an older deaf woman, was "trying to tell me something," as I wrote in my fieldnotes. She touched my then-partner's red bangles, "mimed eating something handful-sized, then made a sort of scrunching gesture with one hand in the palm of the other."

Perhaps these latter movements are what Kendon calls a "ready-made sign," but it was not one I understood, so Jyoti got up to find and show me a discarded pomegranate rind. My partner asked what we were talking about, and when I told her "pomegranates," she said that she had in fact understood, because Jyoti had shown that she was talking about a fruit, pointed to the red bracelets, and "made a sweet face"—which, when I asked, turned out to be a conventional but apparently also quite decipherable sign.[12] It is interesting that my partner understood before I did, even though I had far more experience communicating in natural sign; the immanent relations, one might say, clicked into place for her more quickly. This example illustrates several different strategies Jyoti uses and, more broadly, shows how the immanence of signs in the world makes communication possible even in the absence of conventionally shared signs—although it may take a while, even when the addressee is doing her best.

From a methodological perspective this example indicates that I am not necessarily able to distinguish between the existence of conventional signs and people's knowledge thereof that enables them to produce and interpret such signs, on the one hand, and the existence of social and bodily conventions and people's knowledge thereof that enables them to produce and interpret immanent signs, on the other. What Jyoti first signed to refer to a pomegranate may in fact have been a conventional sign; it also may have been easily interpretable by another person, even if it wasn't conventional to them. Relatedly, I recall seeing a hearing signer in Bodhe trace the shape of a long beard and then hold out his hand as if begging to indicate a *yogi* 'holy mendicant,' which his deaf neighbor seemed to understand, as apparently I did, but I am not sure how conventional this sign was.

What matters here is that not all signs have to be conventional to be produced and/or understood, because of the quality of immanence. My argument here merges Kendon's approach with a practice theory framework. What Hanks (1990:150, parentheses in original) describes as "the process [of typification] whereby actors represent (and therefore understand) themselves and their world" applies both to communicative and other social practices and is grounded in and reproductive of bodily habitus. From this perspective recognition of a sign on the basis of prior familiarity with the sign and recognition on the basis of prior familiarity with the base, the referent, and the world in which both exist are less different than they might seem. Both signers and addressees can use their worldly, corporeal knowledge to produce and interpret movements that may or may not be conventional signs. Put another way, certain forms are immanent in conventional bodily dispositions shared across persons. And in the case of the articulation of immanent, less conventional signs (quadrant 2), signers and addressees work to actualize semiotic relationships that would otherwise remain latent. Moreover, what quadrant a sign belongs to may shift according to the people involved, as with signs that might be immanent for residents but not for me, or conventional and immanent for hearing people who talk regularly with signers while nonconventional but immanent for hearing people who do so infrequently, similar to Kuschel's (1973) analysis of decipherability.

My goal in this book is not always to state with certainty exactly *how* conventional or immanent a particular sign is to a particular person or community. In fact, I have not attempted here to quantify the region's conventional natural signs, though I am confident that there are far fewer than in, say, NSL or Nepali.[13] Instead, I have argued *that* natural sign involves both conventionality (whether immanent or not) and immanence (whether conventional or not) and that these features are critical to its possibilities and vulnerabilities. I seek both to acknowledge and to trouble the line between kinds of knowing—of linguistic convention, bodily convention, shared histories and landscapes—as well as to acknowledge the limits of analytic knowability.[14]

It is also important to recognize that both conventionality and immanence involve affordances and constraints. When signs are conventionally known as linguistic signs, they offer the affordances of all conventional grammatical forms: they are readily available for production and they are easily interpreted. At the same time, signs that are conventional but not immanent must be learned at some point, a kind of constraint based on familiarity, exposure, and indeed willingness to learn. Moreover, the relatively low degree of conventionality in natural sign can itself be a constraint for signers and addressees. Immanence, meanwhile, offers possibilities for both producing and interpreting meaningful signs in the absence of linguistic conventions, but it is also a constraint in that effort is required.

Producing and interpreting immanent signs may not be experienced as "obligate and automatic," Levinson's (2006) description of how users of conventional language experience understanding. Wresting a sign from its immanence in the world to articulate it with the body, or interpreting such a sign, requires work, work that—as detailed in chapter 4—people may or may not be willing to do. While forms motivated by shared experiences of the world need not have been previously encoded in linguistic conventions to be potentially available and recognizable, immanent forms are only articulable and interpretable if you are disposed to experiencing them as such. I am using the concept of disposition here to encompass socialized familiarity and naturalization: a kind of tendency toward acting in a particular way, and the sense that doing so is right, likely, inevitable, one might even say "natural."[15] Doing the work to bring immanent forms into actuality and to understand them both requires, and produces, dispositions/embodied habits.

While explored further in the following chapter, it is worth emphasizing that signing is itself a kind of convention. There are conventional signs; there are conventional combinations of signs; and, critically, there is the convention of signing in the first place. Linguist Michael Morgan (pers. comm.) refers to some places as being more "gesture prone" than others, a phrase I take to include the use of co-speech gesture as well as natural sign and related practices. How do hearing people tend to react when they realize a customer, teammate, neighbor, or stranger cannot hear? What kinds of bodily, affective, cultural, and social habits push people toward using their hands, or toward panicking or ignoring or dismissing someone? In the introduction I wrote about Nonaka's (2007) concept of moral habitus and how it coemerges with shared signed languages as well as Friedner's (2005) analysis of deaf sociality as productive of and produced by the desire to understand and help others understand sign. Sites of emergence and use are thus linked to sites of willingness and desire. How does this play out in Maunabudhuk and Bodhe? I examine in chapters 4 and 5 how a more ambivalent and fragmentary habitus both produces and is produced by a social world in which understanding natural signers is possible, not doing so is also possible, and not trying gets naturalized; the fact that sometimes people can try and still fail to understand further complicates, and reinforces, these dynamics.

CONVENTIONALITY AND EMERGENCE

Meaning is emergent in actual instances—that is to say, through the articulation and reception of particular utterances in particular contexts. Even communicative practices involving conventional language require some labor. Yet more emergent forms of language require additional labor because the schematic grammatical structures (Hanks 1990) and pragmatic patterns that make meaning-making feel effortless are less established, elaborated, or fully shared than in conventional language (Green 2022a).

Some of the hearing people with whom I talked in Maunabudhuk described their sense-making practices in natural sign as "guessing." In July 2010, for example, I had a conversation with one of the local school's headmaster as well as Ganga Limbu, a village official. I wrote:

> The headmaster asked me if the [deaf NSL class] students were now using "standard" (his word) sign language, and I said no, not really, and he said oh they're using the "local" (his word) sign language, and I said yes, and he asked if I understand it and I said some, not completely, and asked if he can, and he said somewhat, that he "guesses" at what they might be saying. I said Ganga understands it well, and Ganga said no, he does the same thing, guesses at what they might be saying, that all the villagers do the same thing.[16]

As with conventionality and immanence, it is impossible for me to say with certainty whether hearing interlocutors like Ganga or the headmaster experienced all signed interactions in the same way, or whether they experienced some interactions as smooth and certain and others as involving more guesswork. Based both on my own experiences of natural sign interactions and on my observations of other people's, I would say that the latter is far more likely—that sometimes natural sign feels like conventional language and other times it does not. I also want to emphasize that deaf signers also have to guess or figure out what hearing signers say—and perhaps even more so, as most hearing signers have much less practice than deaf signers in using natural sign.

From the perspective of linguistic analysis, natural sign utterances at times pattern like utterances in conventional language and are conventional and emergent in similar ways. For example, in everyday usage in Maunabudhuk, the actual referents of natural sign lexical items like OLD-PERSON, BOY/MAN, GIRL/WOMAN, and birth-order terms like JEṬHĀ 'OLDEST' or SĀILĀ 'THIRD-OLDEST' are underspecified.[17] (I use the slash between words to indicate that the glossed sign has a conventional meaning that is represented in English with distinct words.) The sign OLD-PERSON often gets used to talk about a spouse, parent, or parent-in-law; BOY/MAN and GIRL/WOMAN often are employed to refer to specific people; and birth-order terms may refer to a variety of people. In practice, therefore, the addressee must resolve reference on the basis both of the particular context of the utterance and the signer's usual meaning. When Sarawata Limbu signed OLD-PERSON, she almost always was referring to her mother-in-law or father-in-law, while Padma Puri usually was talking about his mother, and Sanu Kumari Limbu about her husband. Jyoti, meanwhile, invariably referred to Sagar with—and only with—the sign BOY/MAN, while when she signed *KĀNCHI* 'YOUNGEST,' she usually meant the sister-in-law with whom she lived, who was the youngest by virtue of her marriage to Jyoti's youngest brother. She would also refer to her niece, however, with the sign *KĀNCHI* in combination with the sign CHILD. At least for birth-order terms, this kind of pragmatic narrowing-down also applies to Nepali as it is spoken in Maunabudhuk and Bodhe.

Natural sign conventions also exist on the level of what might be thought of as syntax, pragmatics, or both. By *syntax* I mean the way that multiple signs together produce a meaning greater, or different, than the sum of their parts because of grammatical relationships; by *pragmatics* I mean the way that multiple signs together produce a meaning greater, or different, than the sum of their parts because of patterns in usage that are not analyzable through grammar but are nevertheless predictable. Whether a specific configuration should be considered syntactic or pragmatic, I leave to other people's analyses. Sign combinations include both sequential and simultaneous articulations, and speech is also sometimes articulated simultaneously during signing, whether sporadically or for long stretches. Descriptions of the grammars of signed languages often emphasize their simultaneous, diagrammatic, and/or spatial properties in contrast to the sequentiality of spoken languages, but it is important to remember that signing also occurs sequentially in time, and speech also involves simultaneity.

Conversation analysis frames sequentiality as expressing a relevance relation across turns (Hanks 2004). In local natural sign sequentiality does this not only across turns but also within them; temporal proximity becomes a primary means of expressing a relevance relationship between two or more referents. To ask who someone is, for example, a signer points at the person and then signs the general wh-question sign Q; these signs are accompanied by a questioning facial expression. It is the sequence of signs, along with the simultaneous facial expression, that makes it clear that a question is being asked and that the question is about the person. *From* whom or *to* whom a relationship might be calculated or named is left implicit and underspecified; an answer might center the original speaker, the addressee, someone else, or no one in particular ("That person is my teacher," "That person lives near your uncle," "That person is married to the woman down the hill," or "That person comes from the village across the valley"). To point at two people in a row, followed by the same question sign Q and accompanied by a questioning facial expression, also enquires about who someone is, or rather who two someones are. Here, however, the sequentiality produces a more specified focal relationship. It is between the two people; the question is who they are *to each other*.

These examples show that conventions exist and that they are more than additive. Pointing at two people in turn followed by the question sign means something different from, though certainly related to, pointing at one person followed by the question sign. It is also conventional that the sign Q follows articulation of the object or relationship being thematized or asked about. Similarly, negatives follow what they negate. Relatedly, reported communication or action is indicated by signing what someone said or did and then pointing to the person who said or did it. In most cases in my video data, the sayer/doer was physically present. In one instance a signer was reporting the utterances of an absent person, and in that case the signer had already established the person as a topic of conversation. She then signed his utterance, followed by a lexical item referring to the person. In neither case—reporting the speech of someone present or absent—does the relationship between what is said and who said it get identified with a lexical item meaning 'say.' Instead the relationship is given by their sequence, with the subject coming second.

The following example exhibits several of the just-described conventions. The signer is a hearing neighbor of Sarawata Limbu and her husband, both deaf. Joking about people getting married or running off with other people, as in this example, is a common local genre in both speech and sign. Of particular note is the neighbor's use of the term *JEṬHI* 'OLDEST' along with the sign GIRL/WOMAN to make reference to Sarawata; as the oldest son in his family, Sarawata's husband is known as *jeṭhā*, so Sarawata, his wife, can be referred to as *jeṭhi*. Also relevant are the use of what seem to be a hypothetical quoted utterance and a hypothetical reported action, with the attributed utterance/action followed by a point to the person to whom it is attributed, who is also the addressee. The hypothetical utterance is also prefaced by a point, so there is some ambiguity in the point's functionality: engaging with the addressee, referring to him, and/or attributing utterance/action. Line breaks are for ease of reading, and the slash between GLOSSES/*italics* indicates simultaneous articulation of sign and speech; note that in this example, the neighbor's spoken words either double what she signs (e.g., pointing at someone to get his attention while saying in Nepali "*yatā* 'this way,'" pointing at someone to refer to him while saying in Nepali "*u* 'he'") or refer to what has been signed (signing "ELOPE" and saying in Nepali "*yaso* 'that'"). While in line 4 it is the woman's spoken intonation that tips me slightly toward marking it as a question rather than a statement ("You are going to . . .?"), the versions function more or less equivalently in this context. Finally, a sign followed by the plus sign + indicates repetition of that sign.

1   Point-husband/*yatā*
     Hey (in speech: **this way**)
2   Point-Sagar/*u* ELOPE/*yaso*
     Sagar's going to elope (in speech: **he, that**)

3   Point-husband *JEṬHI* WOMAN GO-TOGETHER Point-outward,
     with your wife, they're going to run off together.
4   Point-husband COME+/*āune* Point-husband, CRY/*rune* Point-husband?
     Are you going to say, "Come back, come back," and cry? (in speech: **come, cry**)[18]

GUESSING PART 1: HOOKS AND FILTERS

The process of "guessing" described by several hearing people was frequently imperceptible to me. I could only observe people's actions and sometimes learn more about the situation later. One day, for example, I saw Ram Aryal, a hearing man, ask Bal Limbu, a deaf man, a question that consisted of holding up two fingers, making the conventional sign MONEY (the first finger rubs quickly against the thumb of a loosely closed hand), and putting that same hand into a pocket. This last action Kendon (1980b) would call a "characterizing enactment," and I would call a sign immanent in the relationship of bodies, clothing, and money. I interpreted Ram's utterance as a question, which would have been due to a conventional facial expression or head movement, the use of the conventional Q sign, or some combination of these. I had a general sense of the topic, but it wasn't until the following day that I had the opportunity to find out more: the question referred to Bal's two nephews, who had stolen a thousand rupees and run away.

In his utterance Ram did not specify what the number two was quantifying; generally, natural signers use numbers to quantify and refer to persons, animals, days, years, physical objects, and other things. Here, Bal had to figure out that TWO was enumerating people. Those two people were linked with an action through sequential articulation. The action had to be interpreted not as (only) the literal placing of money in a pocket but also as taking money surreptitiously. To understand his neighbor's question, Bal had to connect the directly stated parts of the utterance (TWO, MONEY, PUT-IN-POCKET) to each other and also elaborate on them; doing so would have required familiarity with signing (which he of course had as a deaf signer), with the kinds of elisions made in natural sign, and with the kinds of questions people ask of one another, as well as familiarity with the state of affairs or type thereof (past, present, or future, real or hypothetical) to which Ram might plausibly be referring.

Natural sign is not unique in the way that signers require their addressees to do sense-making labor beyond the uttered signs/words; it is easy to imagine someone saying in English, for example, "Those two, and the money, huh?" But this sort of leanness is typical for natural sign, even in cases where a topic is being raised for the first time, and it is a feature connected to the way that natural sign utterances—and ultimately natural sign itself—are so emergent. The signs act as potential hooks, reaching out into the world. If the addressee chooses, they can participate in what Goodwin (2018) calls "cooperative action"; they can gather those things up and put them together in a way that works. The signs can also be thought of as performing a filtering or narrowing function; here, once the pieces are brought together, through their temporal adjacency, the TWO narrows the possibilities for which money the landlord might be talking about, and the MONEY getting PUT-IN-POCKET narrows the possibility for which TWO the landlord might be talking about. Note that a later sign may narrow an earlier sign's possibilities just as much as an earlier one may narrow a later one's.

Occasionally I was able to observe more directly the process of putting together that I have just imagined for Bal. For example, I witnessed a conversation in which Parvati Khadka, a deaf woman, relayed a series of details: fingerprints, many houses, on the other side of the river. Her son Yug and his best friend, both hearing, together figured out in spoken Nepali that Parvati was talking about going to get her youngest son's citizenship card in Dhankuta headquarters; the fingerprints proved to be the most important key or "clue" as I wrote in my fieldnotes.[19] Another form of guessing, one that requires work from both addressee and signer, involves back-and-forth exchanges to reach clarity. For example, on the road outside the NSL class on a late May morning, Jyoti told me that her younger brother's wife had been drunk while carrying water in a *ḍoko* 'woven basket worn on the back, supported by a strap around the forehead' and had fallen, spilling water everywhere. She used speech accompanied by signs, including a signed depiction of liquid spilling and spreading. I asked using spoken Nepali and signs if this event had happened yesterday or today. I thought she said today, so I indicated a very early morning time by using a flat, extended forearm to point very low in the eastern sky, a conventional way of indicating time. Jyoti corrected me, showing a late afternoon position. Since it was still morning, I realized the event must have happened the day prior to our conversation.[20]

ZONES OF RELEVANCE AND THEIR ABANDONMENT

In several of these examples the signs both create and call the addressees' attention to what Schutz (1970:111) refers to as a "zone of relevance." Paying attention to zones of relevance is an important dimension of understanding natural signers: what domains of life are significant to the utterance at hand? Yet one must also be willing to abandon zones of relevance, or rather, abandon one zone of relevance for another; sticking too closely to one zone can itself impede understanding. For example, one day in NSL class we were going over a chart of illustrated NSL vocabulary that includes many different birds along with a bat. At one point Jyoti grabbed her elbow/forearm with the other hand, made a loose flapping gesture, and then signed "COLD." I began to try to figure out what she was saying in relation to birds and bats, partly because of what we had just been signing and partly because the form of Jyoti's sign resembled, in my mind, a beating wing. Both Sanu Kumari, another deaf natural signer, and Sagar, the deaf NSL teacher, however, immediately understood that Jyoti was talking about something completely different. As Sagar said: "Oh, she's sore in the morning."[21]

Sanu Kumari and Sagar were able to make sense of what Jyoti signed, while I could not, for at least two reasons. First, to them the movement of Jyoti's arms resembled not a beating wing but rather how a person moves around to loosen up stiff joints. Here, resemblance is literally in the eye, and perhaps the muscle memory or mirror neurons, of the beholder. I grew up in subtropical Florida, went to a college with overheated dorms in the northeastern United States, and then lived in temperate Oregon and Northern California prior to doing fieldwork in Nepal; Sanu Kumari and Sagar were both from the area and thus deeply familiar with how local residents feel and move their bodies on cold mornings in unheated houses. Key here are both their experience of the environment obliquely invoked and the fact that movements like stretching are themselves culturally specific and learned (Mauss 1973 [1936]).[22]

Second, both Sagar and Sanu Kumari were willing and able to let go of a close relationship between the referents of the signs we had been making and the signs Jyoti then made, whereas I assumed there must be one. Whether their familiarity with the referent of Jyoti's movements enabled them to abandon the zone of creatures that fly or whether the abandonment of creatures that fly enabled them to recognize what she meant is an unanswered, perhaps unanswerable, question. And what would have happened if Jyoti's signing had no formal similarities, put one way, or perceived resemblances, put another, to the previous signs' forms and referents (birds and bats)? Perhaps if I had not perceived any linkage, I would have been more likely to leave the zone of flying creatures entirely and try to enter into a new one. However, if there had been no such linkage, perhaps Jyoti would not have made her comment in the first place. My instinct is that Jyoti *felt* a similarity in her body between the forms the lesson asked us to make and the movements she would make on chilly mornings to ease her aching joints.

GUESSING PART 2: MISTAKES

In the earlier examples of Bal's nephews and Parvati's citizenship card, I cannot say for sure what the signer intended, but the addressees seemed to figure it out. In the following three examples, in contrast, I had some access to what the signer meant to communicate to the addressee: in the first two examples, because a hearing signer also (probably) spoke aloud in Nepali, and in the third example, because I was independently familiar with the event to which (I believe) the signer was referring. And in each of these examples, some kind of miscommunication occurred, at least from my perspective. The use of two examples where a deaf signer misunderstands and one where a hearing person does is not intended as iconic of the demographics of (mis)understanding. Rather, it reflects that signers who speak at the same time often express the same thing in both modalities, thus making it unambiguous, from a methodological perspective, what was meant.[23]

Krishna Gajmer's hearing older brother, Samman, and Sagar generally communicated well, even toward the beginning of their acquaintance, but there were occasional hiccups. On one occasion in June 2010, Samman asked Sagar where he lived; Sagar, however, thought that he was asking if their homes were similar. As a practice, I would only have made a firm declaration (in my fieldnotes or to Sagar—both of which I did) about what Samman said if I had a definitive way of knowing. In this case, reading back in my notes, I assume that Samman, who frequently used sign and speech at the same time, signed something like "HOME Q?" and simultaneously spoke in Nepali something like "*ghar kahā̃ tapāīko* 'where is your home'?" In this instance the misunderstanding seems to be located in the broadness of the question. The general wh-question sign in natural local sign is underspecified. The question as signed could be translated into English as something like "What about your home?" or "and your home?" Here, Samman clearly intended it to mean "where," as he uses the Nepali *kahā̃* 'where.' It is possible that among local signers that would have been the default meaning when paired with the sign HOME; recall from chapter 1 that Sagar told me that he had asked Krishna, who happens to be Samman's deaf brother, "Where do you live?" with the signs "HOME Q?" For whatever reason, in this instance Sagar interpreted Samman's query not with regards to location but rather as a request for an evaluation of his home's likeness or difference from the home in which we were currently situated.[24]

The Q sign is also implicated in a second example. As discussed earlier, pointing to someone followed by the Q sign means "Who is this person?" while pointing to two people in turn followed by the Q sign means "How are these people related?" During a video-recorded conversation between Padma Puri, a deaf man, and two hearing teenage girls, Shanti and Charu, the following exchanges took place. Here the lines indicate turn-taking, a slash between uppercase gloss and lowercase italics indicates simultaneous sign and speech, and a slash between glosses indicates polysemy or ambiguity. The parentheticals describe nods, pauses, or when I have had trouble hearing the recording, and a verb followed by a place (such as COME-here) indicates the path of motion of the verb. In the translation for line 10, I have written both what the girl seems to have meant, based on her spoken words, and what Padma seems to have understood.

1 Shanti: Point-self Q? Point-Padma Point-self Q?
           Who am I? What's our relationship?
2 Padma: Point-self? (hesitates)
           Me?
3 Shanti: (affirmative nod)
           Yes
4 Padma: (hesitates) Point-left COME-here COME-here
           I came here from over there
5 Shanti: (hard to hear) *ke bhaneko?*
           What'd he say?

6   Charu: (hard to hear) *ke bhayo?*
             What happened?
7   Shanti: *"mero ke parne?"* bhaneko (more that I can't hear)
             I said, "Who are you to me?"
8   Charu: uncle bhannu na . . . uncle, uncle
             Say he's your uncle
9   Padma: *KĀNCHHĀ* 'YOUNGEST' ONE COME
             ***Kānchhā* comes/came this way**
10   Shanti: (gets Padma's attention) Point-self ALRIGHT/FINISHED?
             What she meant: **Who am I?**
             What Padma seems to have understood: **Am I alright?**
11   Padma: (affirmative head tilt) Point-self, ALRIGHT/FINISHED, Point-Shanti
             Yes, I am/we are alright
12   Shanti: Point-self Q/*ma ko ho?*
             Who am I?
13   Padma: ALRIGHT Point-Shanti (affirmative head tilt)
             You're alright

I want to make two observations. First, Shanti did not secure Padma's referential understanding. From her spoken Nepali renderings, it is apparent that she wanted to ask Padma how he would characterize their relationship. Charu articulates a possible answer: he is Shanti's *uncle*, a term of kinship borrowed from English (Turin 2002) that can be applied to people who live in proximity to each other, including of different caste groups, as in this case. Second, despite the misunderstanding, communicative sociality has been achieved and maintained, a topic to which I return in chapters 4 and 5.[25]

Why didn't Padma understand? On the one hand, Shanti's utterance could be said to pattern with the local convention for asking who someone is. As discussed earlier, pointing at someone then articulating Q typically means "Who is this person?" And pointing at two people in turn followed by Q typically means "What is their relationship?" On the other hand, I do not recall seeing any other instances in natural sign of a person pointing to themself followed by the sign Q or to themself and their addressee followed by the sign Q as Shanti does here. In other words, the meaning that she intended, while patterning with natural sign practices, was nevertheless pragmatically unusual, since she was asking about her and Padma's relationship rather than about another person or persons. Padma seemed to interpret her questions, first as asking about himself and what he had been up to (a reasonable interpretation of line 1, albeit one that ignored Shanti pointing to herself, and of lines 2 and 3); and later as asking if she, or the two of them, were alright (another reasonable interpretation of the signs in the second half of line 10).

The third example of misunderstanding is quite different. In late May, Jyoti led Sagar and me to the small house she shared with her youngest brother, his wife, and their two children, a minute or two's walk west from the bazaar. No one was home, so Jyoti walked over to the house next door, where we met her neighbors. During the ensuing conversation, the neighbor's eldest daughter, Nani, told me: "Jyoti said she slept with you the other night, and I told her that was impossible; you're smelly and your teacher is clean." ("To sleep with" here is not a euphemism for sex. I was often asked to sleep at people's houses, even if they lived very close to my own room, as an expression of hospitality and affection. Local residents frequently told me that they were dirty compared to me; in other words, people said this about themselves, not only about other people.) As I discuss more in the following chapters, the kind of evaluation Nani makes ("that was impossible") was not unusual for a hearing person (or a deaf person) to make of (their understanding of) what a deaf natural signer had said. But whereas often the topic of discussion was something about which I could have no independent knowledge, in this instance I was directly involved in the reported event, even if it had happened somewhat differently than Nani was explaining.

Ten days earlier, Jyoti and I had spent time together in the late evening at the home of her *buhāri* 'son's or younger brother's wife.' Jyoti, her *buhāri*, her *buhāri*'s daughter, her daughter's friend, and I had snacked on *kāphal* berries, sweet hard peaches, and Coke, and held an impromptu dance party. Afterward I walked back up a short path and just across the broad dirt road to the house where I rented a room; Jyoti stayed at her *buhāri*'s, as she frequently did. I said as much to Nani: "No, she didn't sleep with me, but we did meet up at *buhāri*'s house. And where I live is close to that."[26]

There are several ways to analyze Nani's evaluation of what Jyoti had said; each one presents different analytic and ethical implications, which I discuss in chapter 5. Here I focus on what I consider to be the most likely scenario: that Nani misunderstood Jyoti and that Jyoti had actually said something about us sleeping in close proximity that night (i.e., in houses across the street from each other), or perhaps that we had been together in the place where she then slept. Both of these possible utterances, along with Nani's version, consist of the same elements: Jyoti; signs such as NIGHT and/or SLEEP; spatial proximity; and me, to whom she probably would have referred with some combination of signs such as FAT, FAIR-SKINNED, and GIRL/WOMAN, and perhaps a sign like SCHOOL, invoking the NSL class, and/or a point toward the community hall where class was held. Nani also correctly placed the narrated event in the very recent past.

In other words, while Nani ultimately misconstrued the story Jyoti told her, she had grasped many of its essential parts. She had, as other hearing villagers described their attempts to understand sign, "guessed" at the relationships among the parts, perhaps even guessed at some of the parts themselves. Perhaps another person might have understood more accurately what Jyoti signed—whether because they were more familiar with signing conventions, with the convention of having to guess, with Jyoti herself, with the event to which Jyoti was referring, or some combination. What I want to emphasize is that the emergent nature of natural sign left room for Nani to do the work of making sense of what Jyoti had said, and in this case Nani was willing to do that work; but the emergent nature of natural sign also left room for the work to go awry.

CONCLUSION

This chapter has answered the previous chapter's call for specificity. Through concrete examples of signs and utterances, it has offered readers a sense of what natural sign is like in this time and place: available and fragmentary, understandable and misunderstandable. In theorizing the concepts of immanence, conventionality, and emergence, I have shown how natural signers produce and interpret signs and utterances that require work. Immanence in particular both complements and complicates chapter 2's account of natural sign's paradoxes, as it highlights how conventionality is itself multifaceted, implicating people's experiences of shared sign forms and communicative practices but also of other kinds of bodily routines and social habits. This account resonates with deaf NSL signers' insistence that communication in natural sign is very much possible, even if limited.

The moments of understanding, misunderstanding, and not-understanding analyzed here provide a scaffold for the final two chapters. As chapter 3 has shown, natural sign offers avenues for meaning-making that do not depend on conventional linguistic conventions. At the same time, making sense of immanent and radically emergent utterances requires more—more attention, more labor, more commitment—than making sense of utterances produced in conventional languages, and this renders natural signers vulnerable in ways that are distinct from users of marginalized but conventional languages. Chapter 4 builds on NSL signers' theories by analyzing the communicative practices of deaf and hearing people using natural sign with a particular focus on attention, willingness, and refusal; chapter 5 further unpacks (mis)understanding as a complex social and analytic phenomenon.

4

Ethics

In 2010, Stella Limbu was fifteen or sixteen years old, a sharp, funny, and kind hearing teenager whose extended family lived in two modest homes: one in the farmlands near the home of two deaf sisters-in-law and another in the bazaar. The latter was smack in between the house where Sagar Karki and I rented rooms and the one where we took our meals, so we saw a lot of each other. When I first arrived in Maunabudhuk, Stella took me under her much-younger wing, and over the next several weeks she often accompanied Sagar and me as we explored the area. The three of us would walk the packed-dirt paths, joking together, visiting deaf residents' homes, and taking breaks to climb the high limbs of sour plum and *kāphal* berry trees to pick fruit (or in my case to watch them do so and then enjoy the literal fruits of their labor). I was struck by the ease with which Sagar and Stella communicated, and even more by her abandonment of speech when in Sagar's company. In general, hearing people who signed would do so only briefly, and I was not the only one so struck by Stella's actions. On one occasion a hearing shopkeeper enquired of Stella, entirely without rancor, "Why aren't you talking?"[1]

There was no obvious explanation for Stella's positive, even delighted, orientation toward signing. None of Stella's immediate relatives are deaf, though like nearly everyone in Maunabudhuk, she knew deaf people. As well as having deaf neighbors, Stella frequently hung out with her best friend in a small snack shop where Jyoti Limbu, an older deaf woman, could often be found doing odd jobs. More important, it seems to me, was the fact that Stella and Sagar genuinely liked each other. They were playful together, joking and teasing in a way that is common among young people in the area. Stella and I also had an affectionate and easy rapport, and the three of us enjoyed spending time together.

Stella's willingness to communicate in sign, and the facility with which she did so, in some senses obscured that very willingness. But watching her and thinking about her has helped me to recognize the traces of pleasure and desire in hearing people's "ability" to sign.[2] Stella's two sisters, one older and one younger, were perfectly amiable with Sagar but neither as interested in nor as adept at directly conversing with him. Moreover, the contrast between Stella's willingness and the kind of refusal with which I opened this book—a woman moving her eyes away from Shrila Khadka as she signed—highlight the critical role played by hearing individuals' sometimes inexplicable orientations toward signers and signing. It is precisely because I do not have a straightforward explanation for Stella's willingness, even eagerness, to sign, nor for her facility in doing so, that I open this chapter by writing about her.

Willingness, refusal, ambivalence, hesitation, eagerness, begrudging attention, curiosity: these orientations toward sign and signers arise from a vast and often unchartable ground comprised of histories of interaction, family relationships and commitments, prejudices against and assumptions about deaf and disabled people, local social hierarchies and affiliations—from love, attraction, dislike, distraction, shyness, shame, and enjoyment. In any given instance it may be impossible to discern why one particular hearing person was so ready and able to communicate in natural sign and another one was so very not. Fully recognizing that I may not be able to pin down the reason for people's orientations, this chapter tracks the socially perceptible actions through which orientations manifest and create effects. As with Stella's joy, or, later in this chapter, Binita's disdain and Samman's quiet care, affect and emotions matter because their expression in actions have concrete consequences.

This chapter therefore pays attention to what disinterest, willingness, or hesitation literally look like and sound like, and to the consequences of other, usually hearing, people's actions on deaf natural signers' everyday participation in communicative sociality. My approach is rooted in a perspective on communication that recognizes the entanglement of pragmatics and metapragmatics—that is, the entanglement of what people (can) do with language and what people think/say about what they (can) do with language (Silverstein 1976; Hanks 1996, 2005a, 2009). The examples and themes in this chapter link back to chapter 1, where I argued that NSL signers' protest against the word *lāṭo* is also a protest against being treated as if they were incompetent or incapable of making sense to and of others. NSL signers theorize intelligibility as a situated quality of particular interactions, not a quality of individual persons. NSL signers also suggest that outside of deaf society, deaf people are particularly vulnerable to being excluded from communicative sociality because hearing people may or may not choose to interact with them in natural sign. This chapter both demonstrates the significance of NSL signers' insights and elaborates on them through fine-grained analyses of interactions in natural sign.

To be clear, not all instances of not-understanding or misunderstanding are the result of unwillingness. In natural sign, as I know from firsthand experience, it is absolutely possible to try, even to try extremely hard, and nevertheless to not-understand or misunderstand. It is nonetheless true that interactions both depend on and (re)produce the ethical orientations people bring to these interactions. Put another way, while interactions are not fully reducible to the effects of orientations, orientations make a difference in whether and how people attend to and understand other people's utterances. That is, instances of communicating in natural sign that hearing people in particular experience as frustrating work to reinforce some of the very orientations that are an often unrecognized factor in creating those frustrating experiences, thus both naturalizing and reproducing the interactional circumstances of natural sign. How any given interaction plays out impacts people's generalized expectations about interacting with deaf signers, and over the long term, can influence the degree to which sign as both form and practice becomes conventionalized and widespread, as suggested in the introduction and chapter 2. Ethical orientations are thus inextricable from the questions of demography and sociolinguistics, affordances and constraints, explored in previous chapters, and not merely an additional factor necessary to make sense of natural sign, both interactionally and analytically.[3]

Some of the variation in hearing (and deaf) people's responses to and evaluations of deaf people and their use of natural sign clustered around particular people and configurations, as I explore more in the following chapter. Sagar consistently, though by no means always, understood and was understood by others, both deaf and hearing. There were times when I would try to tell the NSL class participants something, fail miserably, and watch as Sagar did so with ease. Many hearing people also noticed that it was easy to communicate with him. Among deaf residents, some were socially regarded as sensible people, while others were more likely to be ignored or dismissed, both by deaf and hearing people. But even those deaf signers who were considered effective communicators might not be attended to or understood in a given instance, and even deaf people who were generally thought of as difficult to understand were in fact often understood. To complicate matters further, potential participants' actions and orientations were often seemingly contradictory. For example, on more than one occasion I heard hearing people say in Nepali "I don't understand" but respond in sign to a deaf signer.

TRACKING ORIENTATIONS: EYE GAZE, SIGNS, TRANSLATIONS, EVALUATIONS

Whatever their source(s), orientations get expressed in various actions that also constitute conversational moves. I track orientations through eye gaze (where did people look when someone signed to them or in their proximity?), sign production (what did they sign in response, if anything?), translation (did someone translate what had been signed, or request such a translation? what did that translation involve?), and evaluation (what if anything did people say about the interaction, whether in sign or speech?). These actions—eye gaze, signing (or not), translations, and metalinguistic evaluations—are both part of conversational dynamics and a commentary on them, providing insight into how participants perceive the potential or ongoing interaction. While not unmediated reflections of people's feelings, desires, or opinions, these actions do offer a concrete way to follow how interlocutors engage and disengage in conversation and to analyze the orientations expressed by and realized through those (dis)engagements.

Methodologically, tracking orientations in these ways allows me to attend to the materiality of social interaction and to anchor claims about ethics in observable bodily actions. Moreover, I can review these actions in video recordings from the field. Eye gaze, accompanying shifts in posture, and signing, or its absence, were available both to me and at least potentially to other participants during interactions, as to the best of my knowledge, everyone with whom I worked in Maunabudhuk and Bodhe was sighted. Spoken translations and evaluations were not fully accessible to deaf signers, although they could see that something was being said, and some spoken evaluations were accompanied by facial expressions or gestures. Eye gaze in particular, as both a conversational move and a commentary on conversation, merits further exploration. Attention to the role of sight in deaf practices has played an important role in deaf studies' commitment to understanding, describing, and theorizing deaf sociality in terms of what it involves and entails rather than what it lacks.

In 1912, long before deaf studies as a discipline came into existence, George Veditz, president of the US National Association of the Deaf, famously characterized (sighted) deaf people as "first and foremost and for all time, people of the eye" (cited in Bauman 2008:12).[4] Bahan (2008) writes about a deaf man and his deaf daughter who are able to pick out another deaf man in a crowd by watching how he orients and responds to the visual dimensions and rhythms of a generic urban scene. Father and daughter are able to identify the stranger as deaf because they see and recognize the visible dispositions characteristic of deaf visual practices (Bahan 2008:83). According to Sirvage (2015), such practices also include an implicit commitment to "watching out" for what is happening behind the back of one's interlocutors and informing them as needed.[5]

While these are examples of more paraconversational social actions, sighted signers and sighted speakers also use eye gaze to establish participant frameworks, manage conversational turns, and convey appropriate interest (Goodwin 1981; Bahan 2008; Sidnell 2010). Goodwin (1981) reports that speakers actively monitor their addressees to see if they are watching them. When addressees are not watching, speakers perform particular actions, such as verbal restarts, to "secure the gaze and orientation of" those addressees (Goodwin 2006:118). A similar claim is implicit in Bahan's (2008) work on signers and their addressees. People watch each other and they watch each other watch each other, attributing meaning to what they see of the other person's eye gaze. And in general, conversational participants interpret eye gaze as attention. The object of attention might be a conversational partner, a third party, an object in the environment, and so forth. As Goodwin

(2006:99) writes: "The gaze direction of an actor . . . allows others to make inferences about what the party is attending to"—and in this case those "others" include an anthropologist. The idea that eye gaze is an attentive and agentive act resonates with the conceptualization of aural listening as active rather than passive (e.g., Hirschkind 2006; Marsilli-Vargas 2014; Friedner 2022).

Of course, as any teacher can attest, the eyes may be directed toward a speaker while the mind is directed elsewhere; nor am I claiming that attention can only be enacted or tracked by eye gaze.[6] However, in visual signed communication, eye gaze is not only an important but also a necessary mode of paying attention; the absence of an intended addressee's eye gaze precludes all other possibilities of their engagement: perceiving what has been signed, attempting to understand, actually understanding, asking for clarification, or otherwise responding. Eye gaze is not sufficient for understanding visual sign, but it is necessary, and looking at a signer both signals potential willingness to interact and makes it materially possible to do so. Eye gaze embodies intention to participate in the conversation and makes that intention actionable.

The importance of eye gaze is, moreover, clear to deaf signers. During a conversation with Prajwal Dangol about his educational experiences, he told me that even though he had successfully passed his School Leaving Certificate exam, he hadn't really liked school. When I asked if the problem was communication, at first he said that the teachers could sign just fine. But then he explained that they would "just say the signs that go along with the words," rather than providing conceptually rich explanations or delving into topics deeply. In other words, the teachers would sign in what NSL signers call LONG SIGN, using NSL signs but Nepali grammar, leaving students with only a superficial sense of what was meant, as if I had written this sentence with English words but according to the syntax and pragmatics of an unrelated language. During our conversation Prajwal provided a memorable representation of his response to the teachers' failures to offer him meaningful lessons, using what sign linguists call "constructed action" (Cormier, Smith, and Sehyr 2015:167). As I wrote in my fieldnotes: "He did an incredible rendition of himself refusing to even look at the teachers (and looking like a real punk-ass) once he lost respect for them." This conversation illustrates the link for sighted deaf signers between respect and eye gaze and emphasizes the materiality of language.[7] There are, however, other ways of showing disrespect than failing to look.

A REFUSAL

One July morning in 2010, Shrila Khadka, the deaf woman featured in this book's opening vignette, approached a shop in the bazaar to ask a tailor to make a *cholo*, a type of women's shirt, with some pretty red fabric her family had given her. She signed the item she wanted by twice mimicking the act of tying, once at her left breast and once at the left side of her stomach, and indicated that she wanted the typically long sleeves to have buttons. The tailor, Binita Pradhan, said she didn't understand what Shrila was saying. Other young women hanging out at the shop quickly recognized what Shrila was requesting and translated her utterance into spoken Nepali, signaling referentially and metalinguistically that her signs had meaning (Jakobson 1959, 1960). At this point Binita said that she didn't know how to make a *cholo*, which may or may not have been true.[8]

As with the opening vignette of this book, the question of why some people understood Shrila and others did not is complicated. Binita had not grown up in Maunabudhuk, so perhaps she had less familiarity with natural signing than longer-term residents. However, as discussed in chapter 2, there is no particular reason to believe that there were not deaf people wherever Binita had grown up and, although there are differences across regions, familiarity with natural sign in one place scaffolds one's ability to communicate in it elsewhere. Moreover, Binita, Sagar, and I all rented rooms in the same home, and this particular morning in July was by no means the first, second, or third time Binita was interacting with a deaf signer.

In terms of Binita's reception of this specific utterance, it is important to know that a *cholo* has a very particular design, recognizable to anyone with a passing knowledge of Nepali sartorial habits and certainly to someone who sewed professionally (figure 16).[9] In the language introduced in chapter 3, Shrila's signs were immanent in the shirt as a sociomaterial object. The form she used enacted the sign's base: what hands do when tying a *cholo*. Furthermore, Shrila addressed these signs to a tailor in a tailoring shop, not to a cook in a restaurant nor even to a tailor in some other context, such as at a communal water tap or on a bus. The meaning of her signs was both immanent in and emergent from the articulation of the signs in context. Everything thus conspired to make Shrila's signing interpretable.

One possibility is that Binita did understand what Shrila had signed but responded by saying she had not. People profess not-understanding for a variety of reasons and strategically misunderstand others (Hinnenkamp 2003; Bernstein 2016). Perhaps Binita felt awkward or wanted to distance herself from deaf people. If she understood but said she did not, then in semiotic terms she interpreted the sign in her own mind but produced for others a sign that denied that she had done so, saying in Nepali that she didn't understand.[10] It is also possible that Binita "really" did not understand. As shown in chapter 3, it is possible to try and to fail, as I initially did when Jyoti was signing about pomegranates. Did Binita try and not succeed? Or did she not try in the first place?

In writing about this event, I find it difficult to separate Binita's general orientation toward deaf people from her stated lack of understanding. I saw Binita act in several instances with blatant disrespect for Sagar, using the derogatory term *lāṭo*—and letting her young daughter use it in reference to Sagar—even after we asked her not to.[11] In contrast, I noticed that some village residents adjusted how they referred to deaf people after being asked to do so. I also have a strong memory of Binita addressing Sagar in spoken Nepali with the second-person pronoun *tā*.

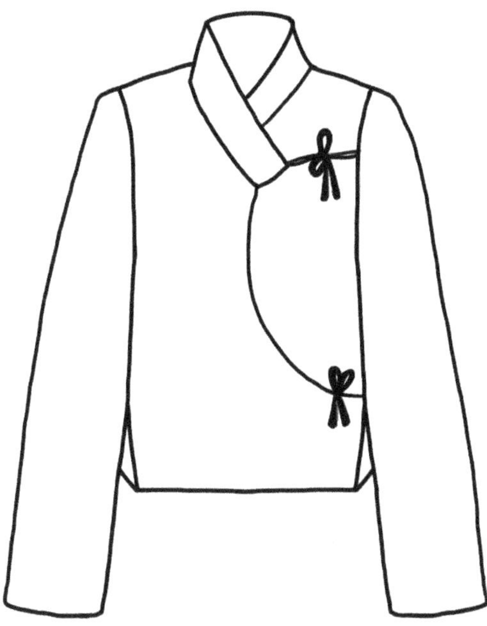

FIGURE 16. A *cholo*: a long-sleeved collared women's shirt that wraps across the torso and fastens with ties on the side. Illustration by Nanyi Jiang.

In everyday speech *tapāī* (or even the more formal *hājur*) is used for strangers of similar age, elders, and people in positions of prestige. The second-person *timi* is used for children, among close friends, and frequently by husbands toward wives. The pronoun *tã* is generally reserved for young children and for insults and was glaringly inappropriate for Binita to use with Sagar, given their roughly similar age, their lack of close friendship, and his position as a teacher. And again, the sign that Shrila used was begging to be understood. Even the most immanent of signs, however, do not simply make sense; someone must make sense of—perceive and interpret—them. To do so requires willingness, and that which requires willingness can be refused.

From one perspective it very much matters whether Binita tried and failed, did understand but pretended not to, or did not try and therefore did not understand. If Binita tried and failed to understand, her failure did not in fact constitute a refusal at all. But her responses did not give any indication that she was trying, and I find it almost impossible to imagine that she could have tried and not understood. Of the remaining two options, the first (understanding and saying otherwise) would constitute an intentional social refusal of Shrila as an intelligible signer. The second (not trying and therefore not understanding) would also constitute a social refusal, as well as a cognitive, embodied, and/or unconscious one, depending on one's view of linguistic processing, decision-making, and the psyche. This kind of not-understanding, in other words, would not reflect the possibilities and constraints of natural sign's semiotics; it would instead constitute a refusal of the very possibility that an intelligible semiotics was present in the first place.

In the scenario where Binita understood but said she didn't, ethics manifests in the social reporting of or response to semiotic interpretation. In the latter scenario, where Binita didn't even try, ethics saturates semiotic interpretation itself—a process that frequently happens below the level of awareness (as with the sentence you are reading now). This analysis deepens the framework and claims of ordinary ethics, in which ethical action is agentive but also deeply habitual and corporeal, as discussed in the introduction. In cases like this one, the line between sense-making as an ethical process and sense-making as a semiotic process becomes so thin that it disappears. The line between ethics and semiotics is similarly obscured—or rather, made particularly clear, which here comes to the same thing—in instances like the book's opening vignette, when hearing people would enact an assumption of unintelligibility with their bodies, announcing "I don't understand" while shifting their gaze away from the signer, thus making it impossible to see what the signer was saying. Other times, people did not necessarily turn their gaze or posture, but they would cease to attend to the signer, their eyes taking on an expression that I came to think of as an eye glaze.

And from another perspective, whether Binita tried but failed, understood but refused to acknowledge it, or did not try does not matter at all. Her stated not-understanding was interactionally indistinguishable from an unwillingness to try to make sense of Shrila. Without additional actions to contradict or nuance her statement of not-understanding, such as signing an answer while saying she had not understood or asking someone else to provide a translation, the effects of (a statement of) not-understanding are the same regardless of the locus of refusal, marking the signer as not-understood and perhaps not-understandable. Both the orientation and the consequences are ethical in nature.

Binita refused to perform the service of sewing a *cholo*—but Shrila could, and eventually did, get her *cholo* sewn elsewhere. More important (for my analysis, if not for Shrila at the moment), Binita refused to engage as a conversational participant. By saying that she had not understood, she refused to constitute herself as an addressee. Given Duranti and Goodwin's (1992:148) argument that "most basically a speaker needs a hearer," Binita failed to ratify Shrila as a signer. Her lack of request for a translation could be interpreted as either a pragmatically neutral move, or as an implication that Shrila was most likely not intelligible to anyone, not just to her. The other girls and women did voice Shrila's request, transforming themselves from overhearers (unaddressed people who nevertheless perceive communication) to animators (people who physically articulate what someone else has communicated), to use Goffman's (1981) terminology. Their animation ratified Shrila as a signer, albeit one who required mediation, within the broader multimodal ongoing conversation, but did not constitute a response to Shrila in sign. It is also important to note that there are not always other people around who are willing or able to provide translation.[12] During my fieldwork, refusals like Binita's were by no means ubiquitous. Hearing people in Maunabudhuk, Bodhe, and other parts of Nepal are often very willing to adjust their communicative practices in interactions with deaf people, shifting from speech to sign, trying to understand. However, refusals such as Binita's were also not unusual.

SHIFTS AND CONTRADICTIONS

On a warm June afternoon in 2010, Sagar and I went to visit Krishna Gajmer, a regular participant in the NSL class, who lived with his older brother, Samman, about fifteen minutes downhill from the bazaar. We followed a steep zigzagging path that led us between fields of thigh-high corn and past bursts of bamboo. Upon reaching the farmhouse, a neat two-story building surrounded by lush flower and vegetable beds, we found Krishna in his family's open-air black-smithing workshop. We settled down for several hours, watching, listening, and conversing as family members and clients came and went; we filmed these interactions for just over an hour. The sequences of exchanges on which I focus here involve Krishna, Samman, their nephew, a neighbor, Sagar (behind the camera), and me. Krishna and Sagar are deaf; everyone else is hearing, including Samman and Krishna's young niece, snuggled into my lap, and a second neighbor, who did not participate in speech or sign in the focal sequences. Figure 17 shows and describes our spatial configuration.

In the following analysis, I focus on eye gaze, sign production, translations, and evaluations to show the instantiation and consequences of shifting ethical orientations. Line numbers refer to the transcribed excerpts in appendix 5 and are complemented by sketched illustrations of framegrabs from the video. I also offer examples from other conversations that confirm or complicate the dynamics present in the conversation at Krishna's home. These additional examples help to provide a broader but also more nuanced sense of how people do, and don't, engage in natural sign conversations in Maunabudhuk and Bodhe.

For much of the time we were there, Krishna and the neighbor were sitting close to each other, often touching casually. Krishna initiated their first recorded linguistic interaction about five minutes into the video: they briefly discuss the knife the neighbor has brought with him to get fixed. Their second on-video exchange comes at Sagar's prodding; he seems to have requested off-camera that Krishna and the neighbor talk. Krishna touches the neighbor on the shoulder, and the neighbor looks at him, making himself an available addressee. Krishna responds with the conventional sign TALK-WITH, shown in figure 18, followed by a point toward Sagar and the general wh-question sign: "TALK-WITH Point-Sagar Q 'so he says we should talk with each other'" (lines 1–6).[13]

The neighbor gives a perhaps paradoxical reply to Krishna's suggestion, signing "SAY" and then the negating sign (line 7). With its lean form this utterance—"SAY

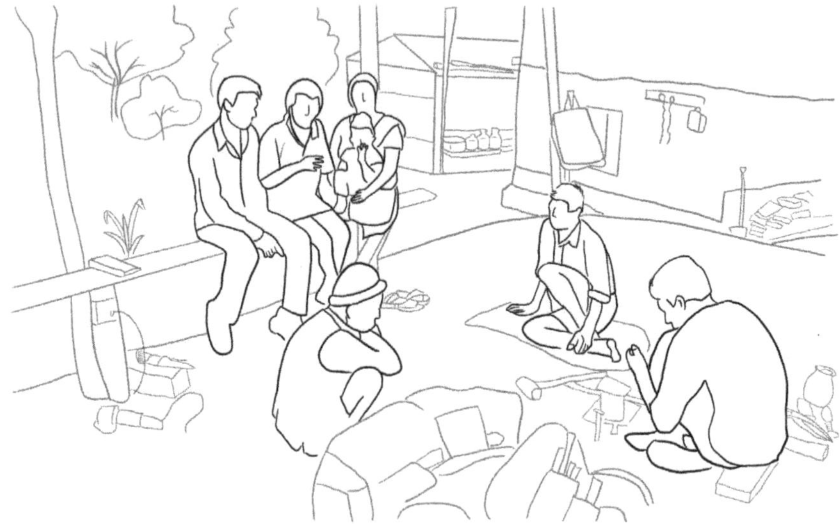

FIGURE 17. In an outdoor blacksmithing workshop, eight people form a rough circle. The neighbor, Krishna, and Mara, with the niece on her lap, sit on a bench; Samman sits on a mat; the nephew works at the forge; and a second neighbor sits near the forge. Sagar is behind the unpictured video camera that recorded this scene. Illustration by Nanyi Jiang.

NEG"—could mean something like "I don't know what to say," on the one hand, or something like "I don't know how to sign," on the other. He may well have felt put on the spot with a video camera recording him. Taking into account the rhythm of the conversation, and his later statements in Nepali that he does not understand much if any sign, however, the neighbor's brief response could also imply that a signed conversation is outside his capacities. Yet in his and Krishna's previous interaction about the knife, and later in the conversation, the neighbor makes it clear that he can sign (even on camera). Regardless of how I interpret it, his utterance suggests that he has understood what Krishna signed—or at the very least, that he is being asked to engage in signed conversation—but also ends the interaction.

During my time in Maunabudhuk, I noticed multiple instances when people said much more explicitly that they couldn't understand yet responded in ways that indicated otherwise. One day, for example, Shrila wanted to get her watch fixed, so she went to a store that sold electronics and waited for a while. Someone told her that the shopkeeper was eating and to come back tomorrow; she waited a little longer and then walked to another shop that used to provide watch repair services but, it turned out, no longer did. She asked the shopkeeper about having her watch fixed, and he said in spoken Nepali that he didn't understand her. But then he pointed her back in the direction of the shop where she had already been. (He would not have known that she had already been there, so he wasn't giving

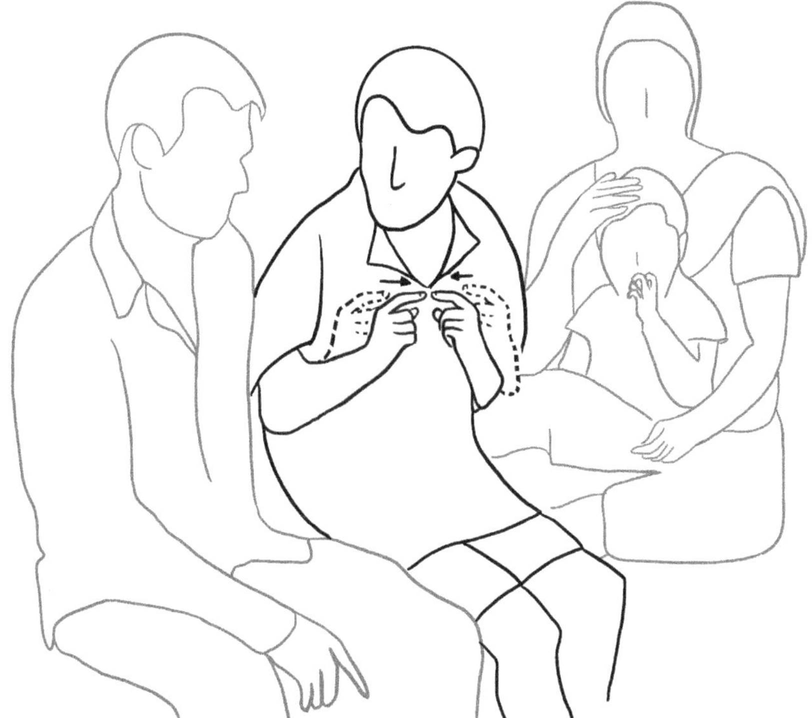

FIGURE 18. Sitting between the neighbor and Mara, Krishna signs "TALK-WITH," two bent index fingers moving toward each other. Illustration by Nanyi Jiang.

her the runaround.) Even though he said he didn't understand, he had understood enough to direct her to a place where he thought she could get the service that she had just requested of him. On another day Shrila and her sister-in-law Parvati were talking to a teacher from a nearby town who happened to be in Maunabu-dhuk. Watching them, I noticed that he sometimes engaged with them and some-times did not, and that out loud he said that he didn't understand anything, despite the fact that he clearly could understand and interact, at least to some degree.[14]

These examples illustrate how at times hearing people say that they cannot understand a deaf person's sign, even when they can, at least in part. Such state-ments are produced in reference to a particular instance of communication and to the ability of the addressee to understand, but they function more broadly as evaluations of deaf signers' general capacity to make sense/be made sense of. Evaluating yourself as having not-understood while responding as having under-stood serves as commentary on the type of interaction going on—the type that is likely to be not-understood, even if in this instance you happened to—and such statements reflect, reproduce, and naturalize the option of nonengagement by potential addressees, even in instances where engagement occurs.

Over the next five and a half minutes, Krishna and the neighbor do not interact. Krishna briefly leaves, then returns to sit on the long wooden bench between the neighbor and me, at which point Krishna, Sagar, Samman, and I exchange signs for about twenty seconds. From our on-camera responses, it appears Sagar was again instructing Krishna to start talking with someone. During this exchange the neighbor looks away and downward, presumably at the forge. Samman is both signing and speaking, so the neighbor's disengagement is from both sign and speech. Indeed, a few minutes earlier I had asked the little girl cuddled on my lap where she attended school using spoken Nepali. She stayed quiet, and both the nephew and Samman teased her about not speaking; the neighbor did not seem to pay attention. It is possible for hearing people to hear speech even if they are not looking at or tuned into a conversation, however, while "overhearing" visual sign requires looking, as discussed in the introduction. Thus the neighbor's potential to become a more active participant in the spoken conversation was not affected by his visual and verbal disengagement in the same way that his potential to become a more active participant in the signed conversation was affected by his eye gaze.

Soon Krishna again signs to the neighbor to report Sagar's suggestion that they interact (line 9). When addressed directly, the neighbor turns and looks at Krishna, who affectionately pats the neighbor's thigh but does not say more. During the same exchange between Sagar and Krishna, Samman visually tracks them, glancing from one to the other. The nephew also looks up from his work to look at Krishna. In other words, while the neighbor looks at Krishna only when Krishna's posture shows that he is directly addressing him, Samman and the nephew constitute themselves with their gaze as overhearers or as unaddressed but ratified participants—people who could be recruited as addressees (Goffman 1981).

Following this exchange, the neighbor returns to looking at the forge, and I ask Krishna about the neighbor. Then Sagar, Krishna, and I engage in a lighthearted discussion about whether the two men present who are Chhetri (a "high," historically dominant caste) wear a sacred thread across their torsos. Sagar and the neighbor are Chhetri; neither wears the thread. During this minute of interaction Samman again visually tracks the conversation, which takes place primarily in natural sign with a few NSL signs. The nephew is engrossed by his own work and does not visually attend to the signed conversation. The neighbor gazes at the forge. I have been asked if the neighbor might have been avoiding the conversation in order to not talk about caste. Despite tensions, people in Maunabudhuk joke about caste and ethnicity across caste/ethnic lines (indeed, I initiated the jokes in this sequence, reflecting my socialization into local humor and conversational practices), and later the neighbor joined in the fun. Figure 19 illustrates the contrast between the neighbor's and Samman's eye gaze.

About a minute later, Krishna again directly addresses the neighbor, who turns to look at him (lines 11–12). At this point I inquire in spoken Nepali, "*bujhnubhayo* 'Did you understand'?" The neighbor replies, "*ma ta hātko ishārā*

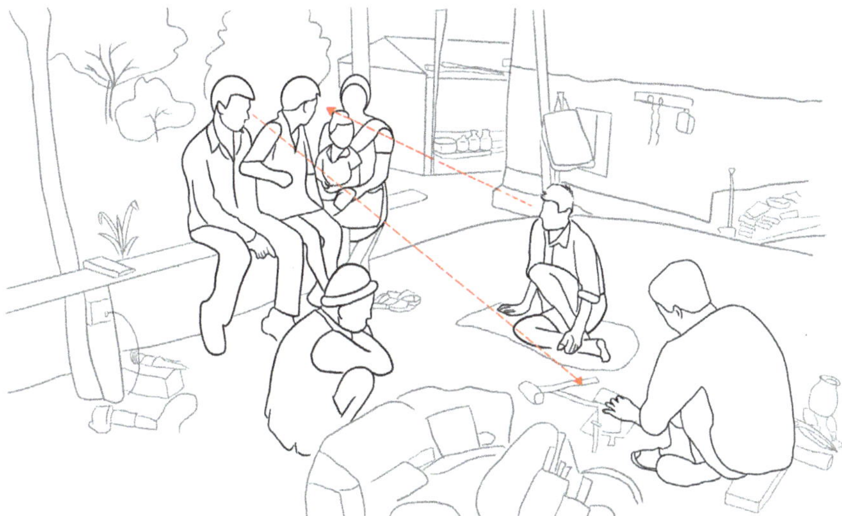

FIGURE 19. In the outdoor workshop the neighbor, Krishna, Mara, the niece, Samman, the nephew, and the second neighbor sit in a circle. Arrows indicate the direction of the neighbor's gaze, at the forge, and Samman's, at Krishna. Illustration by Nanyi Jiang.

ta bujhdina ta 'I don't understand hand signs'" to which Samman responds, "*tyo bāni ho* 'It's a habit'" (lines 13–15). There is a striking convergence here between Samman's invocation of *bāni* 'habit' and the notion of habitus, discussed in chapter 3, as both productive of and produced by engagement with signing; like NSL signers' characterizations of natural sign, comments like this one have informed my analysis.

The neighbor's spoken claim in line 14—"I don't understand sign"—offers a general response to my question "Did you understand?" But in this instance he hadn't given himself the opportunity to understand; he had mostly been staring at the forge. This moment exemplifies how people's orientations, actions, and evaluations are intricately linked. The nephew's eye gaze, meanwhile, shifted as he alternated between watching people sign and attending to his blacksmithing work. People frequently (must) do more than one thing and orient to more than one ordinary ethical project at a time (Lambek 2010:23). In some instances these orientations require shifting hierarchical relations among potentially competing demands (Venkat 2017). This plays out in interactions on a microlevel. In a video taken at the home of Sarawata Limbu, a deaf woman, she is visually and manually engrossed in washing the dishes, but she looks up immediately when someone else begins to sign. Her hearing mother-in-law's attention is also divided between interacting with the other adults present in both sign and speech, and caring for her grandchildren. Sarawata was being a hard-working daughter-in-law and also a deaf signer attuned to signed communication; her mother-in-law a caring grandmother and an engaged host; similarly, Krishna's nephew was working for his family's livelihood and being a younger relative of a deaf uncle.

Soon after Samman's statement about habit, I urge in a mixture of NSL and natural sign that Krishna repeat himself; he does so, signing in natural sign, "SACRED-THREAD THROW-AWAY 'you've thrown away your sacred thread'" (lines 23–25). This time, the neighbor takes a more active role by asking, "*ke bhaneko* 'what did he say'?" (line 27). This short request for translation acknowledges that the neighbor has not understood but that others surely have. Between Samman and the nephew, who is now alternating between attending to the forge and engaging in the conversation, a translation is offered amid much laughter (lines 29–35). Krishna begins to sign again, and now all participants ratify him as a signer, with the neighbor and the nephew both tracking the conversation visually.

A closer examination of Samman's responses shows that even people who strongly orient toward communicating in sign do not always understand. He says to the neighbor that understanding is a habit, and another occasion I asked him directly "*purai bujhnuhunchha* 'do you understand completely' [what Krishna signs]?" He answered that he did, explaining that as they have been talking since Krishna was small, the family understands everything he says and vice versa.[15] Yet Samman fumbles at first when he tries to translate (lines 29–35). In the previous sequence of turns we had used a few NSL signs, and Samman was not accustomed to signing with Sagar or me. Taken alone, then, his hesitation might simply be a matter of unfamiliarity. But I observed other instances when someone's inability to understand or translate specific utterances contradicted their more general statements about always understanding. For example, during a summer afternoon at Sarawata's house I had the chance to chat with her hearing neighbor and relative, Kanchi. I asked if Kanchi understood everything Sarawata said, and she said yes. Later, however, when Sarawata was talking and I asked what she had said, Kanchi replied that she didn't know, that she hadn't understood.[16]

Such contradictions invert the times that people say they don't understand but respond in a way that indicates at least partial understanding. And similarly to how such cases index a general skeptical orientation toward the possibility of making sense in sign, cases such as Samman's and Kanchi's index a speaker's general orientation toward the signer as intelligible. In both of these instances, and in others wherein hearing people articulated a position of understanding, the relationship between the speakers and signers involved kinship, affection, and/or frequent interactions, and it is not surprising that the hearing people would both generally understand and evaluate themselves as such. That in a particular instance they nevertheless found themselves unable to understand further demonstrates the contingencies of natural sign; understanding is not guaranteed, even when the addressee is willing to engage.

Less than thirty seconds after the translation, the neighbor initiates a turn for the first time. Krishna is currently talking with Sagar, so Samman gets his attention

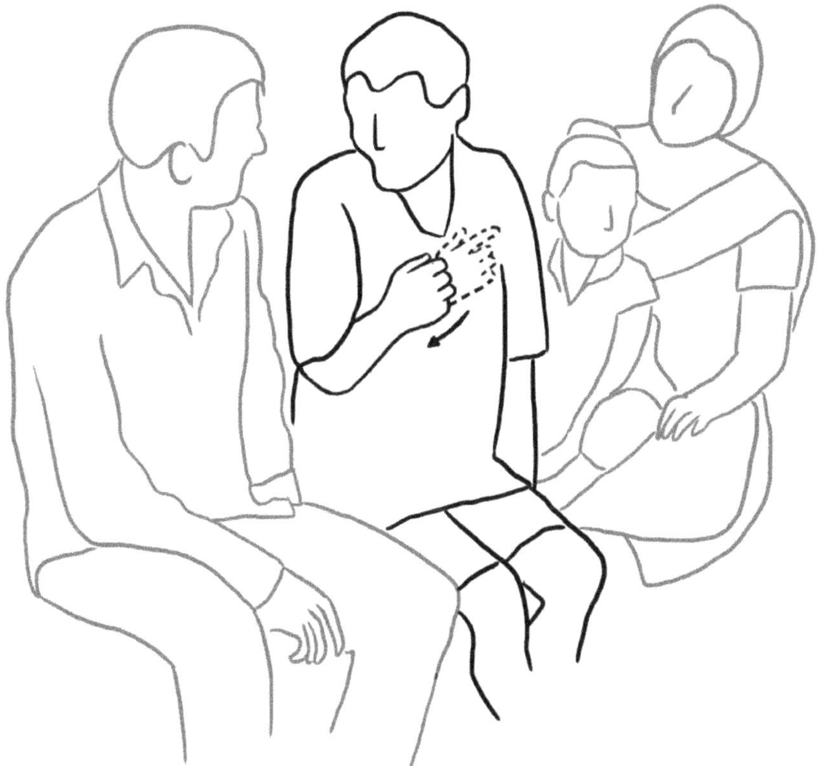

FIGURE 20. Sitting between the neighbor and Mara, Krishna signs "SACRED-THREAD," a forefinger tracing diagonally across the chest. Illustration by Nanyi Jiang.

(lines 36–39). The neighbor repeats himself, signing "SACRED-THREAD NEG 'I don't wear a sacred thread'" (line 40). These signs, and their order, conform to conventional natural sign practices; SACRED-THREAD, shown in figure 20, is also immanent in prescribed caste practices. Then Krishna and the neighbor take turns affirming that while the neighbor has thrown his thread away, the neighbor's older brother still wears his (lines 41–51). The neighbor signs with what appears to be ease, despite his previous protestations of inability.

From this point on, the conversation gets progressively sillier, with Samman teasing Krishna that he should wear a thread and not eat pork. Prescriptively, such actions are expected of Chhetris but not Dalits, so Samman is joking that Krishna should act as if he were Chhetri rather than Dalit. Then Sagar, off-camera, asks if the neighbor eats pork. While the neighbor briefly disengages from the conversation, when Krishna again turns to him, he looks back. Perhaps because of this reengagement, without being asked Samman translates what Sagar just signed into Nepali. In natural sign the neighbor confirms that he does eat pork,

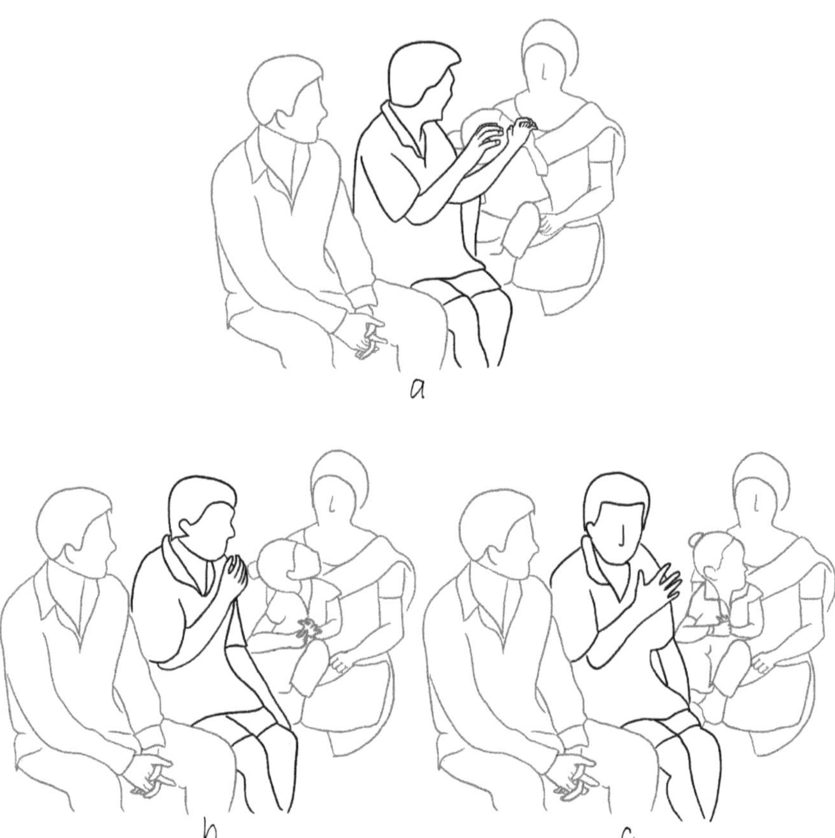

FIGURE 21. Krishna signs "DOG EAT NOT" as the neighbor and Mara watch: (a) two curved hands face outward to sign "DOG"; (b) his loosely closed right hand moves to his mouth to sign "EAT"; and then (c) the same hand, now open, rotates at the wrist in the negating sign. Illustration by Nanyi Jiang.

as well as buffalo (both normatively avoided by Chhetris). He then visually follows an exchange between Krishna, Sagar, and me, in which Sagar jokingly accuses Krishna of eating dog (lines 53–55), which Krishna firmly denies (figure 21). The neighbor understands and successfully intervenes in this exchange, signing with an impressively serious face, "DOG EAT Point-self 'I eat dog'" (line 56; figure 22). This claim is met with raucous laughter.

Then, while Samman in his thoughtful way begins to talk in spoken Nepali about a caste group in India that he had heard eats dog, the neighbor actually continues to banter in sign rather than engage in spoken conversation. He uses a distal point to indicate somewhere far from here. Krishna makes sense of this vague point within the context of the conversation and offers a different sign for

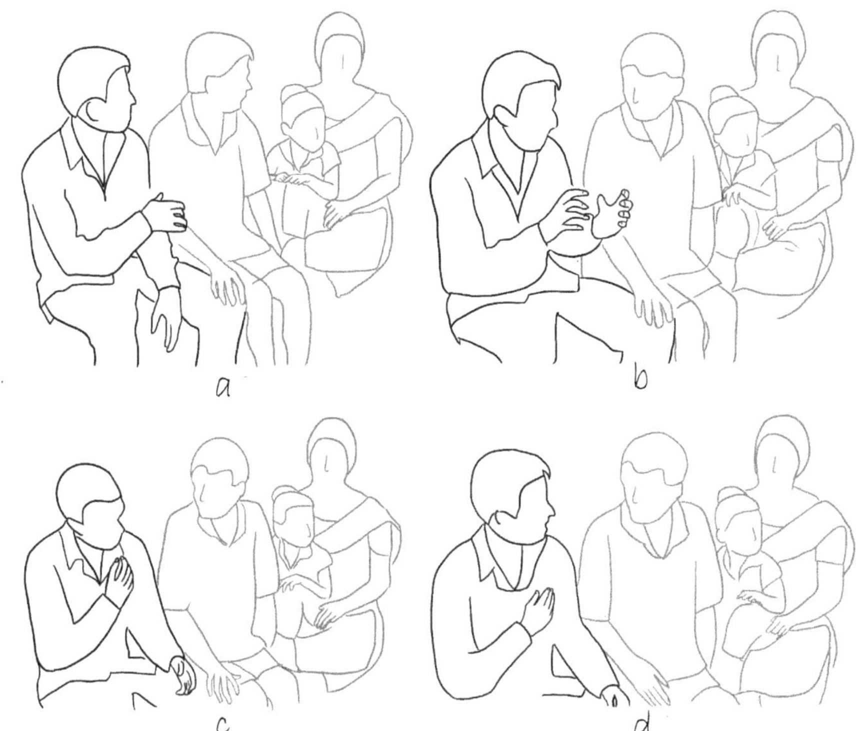

FIGURE 22. The neighbor (a) gets Krishna's attention by touching his arm; (b) signs "DOG"; (c) signs "EAT"; and (d) touches his own chest to indicate himself. The head tilt coarticulated with EAT functions as an emphatic. Illustration by Nanyi Jiang.

ABROAD. Once he uses a flat hand, but on the video it is hard to see how many fingers are extended, and once he uses a flat hand with thumb, pinky, and possibly first finger extended. This second articulation may be borrowed from the NSL sign AIRPLANE, or it may be a local sign. The neighbor takes up the sign with a flat hand, all fingers extended, the handshape I associate with ABROAD as generally signed in Maunabudhuk and Bodhe (lines 65–67, figure 23).

When the neighbor's sign for a horned animal, specified in spoken Nepali as an ox, inspires Krishna to repeat the sign questioningly, the neighbor uses spoken Nepali to request assistance from Samman, who provides it (lines 69–72). The neighbor then describes the slaughtering technique employed abroad, using both a contrasting negative ("they don't cut them like this on the back of the neck") and a signing technique known as "body partitioning" (Dudis 2004): his neck becomes the neck of the animal, while his hand becomes the knife (lines 73 and 75).

This extended example, along with the additional vignettes, reveals the complex, shifting, sometimes subtle and yet deeply consequential relationships between participants' orientations toward signing and the interactional unfolding

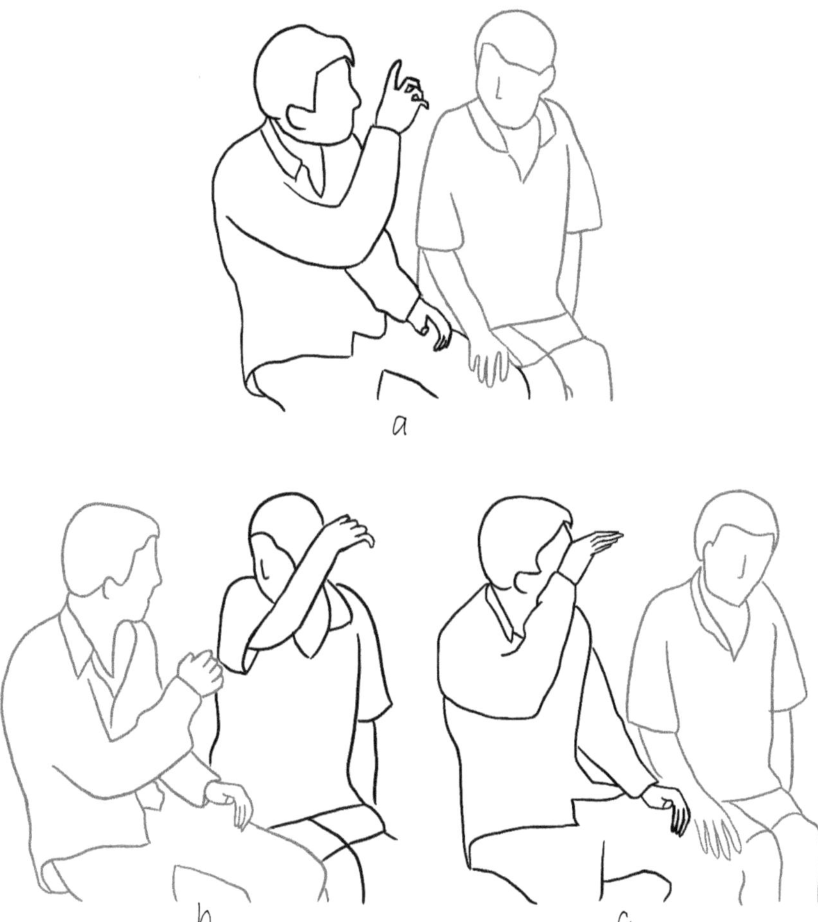

FIGURE 23. (a) The neighbor points up and to his left to indicate somewhere far from here; (b) Krishna offers a version of the more conventional sign "ABROAD," a flat hand with some fingers extended, held high and moving away; (c) the neighbor takes up this sign with a flat hand with all fingers extended. Illustration by Nanyi Jiang.

of conversation in a given context. The neighbor signs that he can't sign, or perhaps that he doesn't know what to sign, and then renders himself a nonparticipant by visually disengaging. Later, he says in Nepali that he doesn't understand; but he hasn't been watching, so how could he have? When he finally joins in, it turns out that he can respond to questions, make jokes, learn new lexical items, talk about actual and counterfactual situations, and take turns appropriately. Samman, meanwhile, embodies and articulates how willingness is both an orientation and a kind of habitus, even if he doesn't understand every single utterance, in part because of the use of some NSL. His eyes move steadily from one party to the other during nearly every signed exchange, adjusting the direction of his sightline slightly in accordance with who was signing. He only occasionally looks down during someone's conversational turn. The nephew alternates between attending to the conversation and his blacksmithing labor.

In both Samman and the nephew, an underlying orientation toward Krishna as intelligible is apparent, as is the materialization of that orientation in eye gaze, sign production, metalinguistic evaluations ("it's habit") and (attempts at) translation. More broadly, these instances show that while refusals by potential interlocutors to engage can deny deaf people the role of signer and the social production of intelligibility, willingness to engage ratifies deaf people as signers and addressees, and produces communicative sociality through ongoing conversation.

BEYOND LINGUISTIC SIGNS

In this chapter's analysis of how hearing people orient toward deaf people and signing, I have thus far focused on overtly linguistic exchanges. Here I turn to an interaction without signs that also recalls how deaf NSL signers talk about the importance of teaching other deaf people to care for themselves in bodily terms (chapter 1). On a late-May evening Sagar and I were walking down the main bazaar road in search of Jyoti Limbu. We found her at her *buhāri*'s restaurant (the one owned by Stella's best friend's mother), where she often worked. In the restaurant there was an older man dressed in tattered clothing. Jyoti's *buhāri* said that she had given him food and that he wanted a place to sleep for the night but that she was closing up shop and he couldn't stay there. I asked who he was, and a few young men walking by said that he was from Dadabazaar, a village an hour or two away. There was debate as to whether or not the man was deaf, but one hearing woman definitely said he was; indeed, the man did not sign very much, but when he did interact, it was in sign, not speech.

Later that evening the older man showed up at the home where Sagar and I, and a few young hearing women who were staying in the bazaar to take exams at the local high school, ate dinner every night. I told my friend who owned the home and cooked that I would pay for the older man's dinner, and she agreed. Those of us who regularly ate there washed our hands as usual; it is even more unthinkable in Nepal than in the United States that eating would proceed without hand washing. Before the old man ate, one of the young women from out of town brought him water to wash his hands, an act that struck both Sagar and me as surprisingly respectful.[17] By bringing the old man water, the young woman made, and perceptibly signaled, a presupposition that he would know what to do with it and that he was competent in the social norms of cleanliness. Using Keane's (2016) framework, the young woman's actions afforded him the opportunity to demonstrate his competency and embeddedness in sociality. Using Goodwin's (2018:268–269) terminology, the man acted on the substrate of the water offered by the young woman, interacting with the young woman and with his environment in meaningful and valued ways.

Whereas the previous examples involve participation in or exclusion from overtly communicative sociality, this example involves sociality without explicitly linguistic communication. It shows how the two are intimately related, as NSL signers know, and shows the impact of what people assume about others on the potential agency of those others to act.

CONCLUSION

This chapter has demonstrated the complexity and the consequences of hearing people's varying orientations toward sign and signers and the actions they take in conversational settings (summarized in appendix 3). Some people, like Samman, are willing and attentive participants in signed conversations. Others, like the neighbor, are more ambivalent, while still others, like Binita, are largely uninterested in making an effort to understand. Individuals' orientations can and do shift, both within and across interactions, sometimes in contradictory ways. Some of these contradictions no doubt arise from the fact that people are involved in more than one ethical project at a time (Lambek 2010:23; Faubion 2011, cited in Venkat 2017). Relatedly, some seeming contradictions can be resolved by distinguishing between hearing people's general orientations toward signing and signers and their specific orientations toward a particular deaf person or a particular conversation/utterance.

More broadly, I suggest that there is an intricate feedback loop among the affordances and constraints of natural sign, people's accumulated experiences of ease and difficulty using it, and the array of possible orientations and actions they perform during conversation. This loop is a concrete exemplar of the proposition that metapragmatics are also pragmatic and pragmatics are also metapragmatic; that what people think can be done with language affects what can/does get done with it, and what people do with language affects what they think can be done with it (Silverstein 1976; Hanks 2005a:230). And these relationships are complex and not predetermined. The affordances and constraints of natural sign shape experiences that shape orientations that shape actions that shape experiences that shape, and create, affordances and constraints. Put more concisely, the fact that people expect that they may (not) understand affects whether or not they (put in the work to) understand. Willingness plays as important, if not more important, a role as the affordances of conventionality and immanence, yet willingness is not a full guarantee that sense-making will occur. While sometimes hearing people refuse to understand, at other times they try and are unable to do so. At the same time, self-evaluations of not-understanding, perhaps particularly when coupled with evidence that understanding has been reached, reinforce that not-understanding is not only a possible semiotic outcome but also a socially expected and accepted one. They reproduce and naturalize a social field in which natural sign is only sometimes attended to and understood.

The assumptions someone makes about understanding someone else and the social-semiotic process of trying to do so (or not) are inextricably entangled, not only with each other but also with how natural sign's semiotic structure leaves room for, and requires the work of, interpretation. In the language of this and the previous chapter, in many ordinary encounters the demands of immanence and emergence mean that the line between semiotics and ethics vanishes. The affordances and constraints that make natural sign so paradoxical are not only material and semiotic, they are also ethical and interactional. Returning to NSL signers' concerns with the way that deaf people get both thought about and treated, deaf-hearing interactions in natural sign may challenge, upend, or reinforce for hearing people the figure of the deaf person as *lāṭo*, a person who does not make sense, especially when the hearing person treats them as such in the first place.

By focusing on hearing people's actions, this chapter has run the risk of over-stating deaf signers' dependence on hearing people. Deaf people are profoundly agentive in their own lives, as these everyday examples have in fact shown. Krishna addressed his neighbor with signs, the older deaf man was in Maunabudhuk in the first place, Shrila approached a tailor to get a shirt sewn and sought to get her watch fixed. While both hearing and deaf people live in worlds comprised of others, it is important to recognize the asymmetry between the people whose ethical orientations have the most impact and the people most impacted by those orientations. The opening vignette of this book shows that a hearing person not-understanding a deaf person may provoke mild censure from other hearing people, but it is unlikely to have lasting or profound consequences for the person who has not-understood. In Maunabudhuk and Bodhe it is primarily what hearing people do and assume others can do that has concrete effects on deaf people's participation in particular interactions and their overall socially evaluated intelligibility as persons. When hearing people do not engage, the effects range in their immediacy and impact, from failing to provide a deaf customer with service to stymying the potential emergence of a more conventional signed language (as discussed in chapter 2), from refusing to look at someone's invitation to tea to disbelieving what deaf signers report about their own lives (discussed in chapter 5).

This chapter has explored the contradictions of natural sign by analyzing the multiple, often contradictory orientations and actions (hearing) people take with regards to natural sign. Those actions include indications of (not) understanding and translations. The final chapter unpacks more fully what translations as well as evaluations of understanding do, what they entail, what they show, and what they conceal, both in conversation and in analysis. In doing so, I return to the entanglement of fieldwork and analysis, not to disavow empiricism but rather to be as empirical as possible. This final chapter delves into the complications and paradoxes of ethnographic research, accusations of lying, and a peculiar dynamic in which Sagar and hearing village residents were often more suspicious of deaf residents' stories than I was.

5
___

Understanding

One afternoon in May 2010, I walked with Jyoti Limbu, a deaf woman, to one of the communal water taps just off Maunabudhuk's main road. A small group of hearing women, teenage girls, and children were taking turns filling up their plastic and metal containers, and I hung back to watch the interactions between Jyoti and her neighbors. While the hearing people present did not ignore Jyoti or refuse to interact with her, she did not appear to be able to follow the casual spoken banter passing between the waiting women, and no one translated it for her.[1] At one point a teenage girl asked Jyoti about her new *pote* 'bead necklace,' bracelet, and haircut, and another woman—the owner of a shop in the bazaar— also interacted directly with her. Earlier in the day, the same woman had asked me in a very friendly manner if I understood Jyoti's *kurā* 'talk.' I replied that I did in part and asked the same of her; she said some. When I asked the woman at the tap what Jyoti had said, however, she replied with the phrase *ke bhanchha, bhanchha.* This phrase literally means 'she says what she says,' where the Nepali verb *bhannu* 'to say' from which *bhanchha* is derived includes both sign and speech, like the English *to say* in this book.[2]

In the context of writing about "belief" in Nepal, Pigg (1996:181) renders an idiomatic translation of this "dismissive little remark": "What does it matter what [she] says?" The phrase *ke bhanchha, bhanchha,* in other words, has a far more negative connotation than phrases like *bujhdina* 'I don't understand' or *bujhina* 'I didn't understand'—phrases that hearing people sometimes utter in response to a signer's signs, as discussed in chapter 4. To be sure, statements about not-understanding do not necessarily accurately reflect whether someone has in fact understood a signer, as when people say they don't understand and yet respond in sign in a way that shows they did. In the utterances *bujhdina* 'I don't understand' and *bujhina* 'I didn't understand,' the first-person pronoun (*ma* 'I') is formally dropped but grammatically present through conjugation. Thus, although social responsibility for failed sense-making accrues to signers, not their addressees, when someone states "I don't understand," the grammatical subject "I" at least offers the possibility of tempering that dynamic.

The phrase *ke bhanchha, bhanchha* is unambiguously dismissive across multiple possible conveyed meanings. The phrase might indicate that the speaker has not understood what has been signed, in a way that implies that either the signer in particular or sign more generally is not someone or something that can be understood; in this sense it functions similarly to an explicit statement of not-understanding that is not accompanied by any contradicting indication of understanding such as a signed response, but with an ever more derogatory flavor. As a direct response to a question about what had been signed, *ke bhanchha, bhanchha* could also imply that while the speaker understood what was said, they did not consider it worth repeating, with the further unspoken suggestion that such was the case for most or all of what that particular signer said more generally. The phrase could also indicate that while the speaker could "make sense" of what had been said on a referential level, it didn't "make sense" in the more colloquial meaning of the English phrase: that is, as something that clearly related to the ongoing context and contributed to the conversation. Without saying so explicitly, the phrase conveys a follow-up question: "If this doesn't make sense, how or why would I respond (or translate)?"

Like the previous chapter, this final chapter analyzes signed interactions among deaf local signers, their hearing families, neighbors, and friends, and Sagar Karki and me. My focus in chapter 4 was on identifying and theorizing ethical orientations, their relationship to how and whether hearing people are willing to engage with deaf signers, and their consequences in interactions. Here I seek to further complicate and nuance what *understanding* means, as both social and analytic processes. What counts as understanding? How do understanding and translation relate to one another? What is the role of misunderstanding? How do misunderstandings simultaneously render deaf signers as intelligible but unreliable? Among other ideas, I suggest that not-understanding may not represent a totalizing state of incomprehension; instead, it can result from an inability to figure out the relations among parts of an utterance that have been understood. Social articulations of not-understanding (that are not contradicted by other signals) may thus conceal partial understanding. And similarly, as when people understand parts and put them together in a way that does not match a signer's intended meaning, stated understanding, responses, or translations may conceal misunderstanding.

Even more than the previous chapters, this chapter portrays some of the difficulties encountered and endured by natural signers in their everyday lives, difficulties that signers did not experience evenly. Some natural signers struggle more than others, and this is true even when they are engaged with people who try to understand them. While in the field, and while writing this book, I have wrestled a great deal with how to think and write about such differences. How can I account for complex biographical histories of people in their thirties, forties, fifties, and sixties, and for possible corporeal, neurological, and psychiatric differences, let alone their entanglement? I am cognizant here of scholars' arguments that language deprivation and communicative neglect can produce developmental and psychiatric disabilities (e.g., Humphries et al. 2016; Kushalnagar et al. 2020). At the same time, I am wary of making armchair diagnoses and hesitant to assume definitively that if deaf natural signers have additional disabilities, they must have been caused by their communicative situations; I believe such an assumption also risks further stigmatizing deaf people with multiple disabilities. I do not have easy answers; as I wrote in the introduction, I am committed to messiness, uncertainty, and a deeply relational approach to sociality, and that guides me here as well. Later in this chapter, I ask what being treated over and over as if you don't make sense does to a person. My wording is purposefully open-ended; some readers may answer this question in terms of language deprivation, and some may answer it through other concepts, experiences, and frameworks.

Related analytic and ethical issues manifest in what might first seem like highly technical matters. Natural signers have a precarious relationship to language as most people think about and use it. When they talk, with other deaf people and with hearing people, what counts as language and what counts as interaction?[3] In asking this question, I return to the affordances and constraints of natural sign. In chapter 3, I emphasized that in natural sign conversations people must put together parts, the relationships among which are often established by grammar in conventional language conversations. In chapter 4, I analyzed how people's orientations toward signers and signing impact their willingness to do that kind of putting-together work. This chapter analyzes a range of situations to further interrogate how ethics impacts reference, and how reference—whether it is understood, misunderstood, or not-understood, and whether or not it is metalinguistically framed as such—impacts how people orient toward signers. Whereas in the previous chapter, the primary examples highlighted hearing people at least sometimes willfully refusing to understand (by looking away or by not making sense of immanent signs), the examples here also reveal people trying and misunderstanding, coming up with conflicting interpretations, or not-understanding at all. If by definition communicating in natural sign is profoundly contingent, and if in interactions between deaf and hearing people the latter frequently have less experience with natural sign (as it is not their primary mode of communication), how do the people with whom I work, and I as a writer, account for those contingencies and their consequences?

This chapter necessarily attends closely to the role that fieldwork played in shaping the very dynamics and phenomena I was and am invested in understanding. I study interaction, and I do so through interaction. Reflecting on her work with signers in Mexico, Hou (2020:667) writes that "the research process itself" plays "a complex role" within the very interactions that researchers analyze. The particularities of my fieldwork—including my presence as a researcher, my imbrication in the NSL class, my ethnographic methods, and my personality traits—are by definition inextricable from what I describe and analyze in this book. Many anthropologists and other scholars have argued that all research—including in disciplines that prize objectivity—shapes the object of study. One of my goals, throughout the book and especially in this chapter, is to recognize and describe that shaping.

I wrote the following passage very early on in my stay in Maunabudhuk: "[Today Parvati] got very upset about a woman she saw walking by and both Sagar and I thought she was saying very clearly that that was her daughter but both yesterday and today a hearing woman insisted that she only has three kids, all sons. It's strange when the veracity of your statement rests in your neighbor's hands . . . not testing one [person's] word against another but more testing one interpretation of those words against another's 'facts.'"[4] Similarly, when a signer told me a story about her own marriage (or so I thought), I asked hearing people to help me sort out what (I thought) she had said. On the one hand, asking hearing people what someone had signed was important both socially and methodologically; as someone new to the area, doing otherwise would have been both arrogant (assuming that I could understand better than they) and impractical (ignoring their potential assistance). At the same time, asking for hearing people's input frequently provided another layer (or two or three) of material to sift through in trying to understand not only the utterances in question but also the broader social dynamics that produced their articulation, reception, and evaluation.

If I received answers that conflicted with what I understood a signer to have said, how might I account for those discrepancies without dismissing deaf signers' own utterances *or* hearing signers' competencies and background knowledge (surely greater than my own) *or* the frequent gaps I observed between deaf and hearing signers? What would different approaches entail? The next section addresses these questions directly.

JYOTI, AGAIN

In chapter 3, I described how a hearing neighbor of Jyoti Limbu, who is deaf, reported to me that Jyoti told her that she and I had slept together (in the sense of sleeping in the same place; not a euphemism for sex) and that the neighbor told her that was impossible because of a perceived difference in our statuses, expressed in terms of cleanliness. This example served to illustrate the profoundly emergent quality of natural sign as well as important consequences of that quality: addressees are called upon to figure out the relationships among parts and therefore addressees may do so incorrectly. In her description to me of what Jyoti had said, Nani, her neighbor, demonstrated that she had in fact mostly understood her; she got many of the elements right, but she put them together in a way that did not match what I believe Jyoti actually was trying to get across. I explained that this was an unusual case, because I was familiar with the event to which I thought Jyoti was in fact referring, a recent impromptu evening of eating and dancing in a relative's home where Jyoti sometimes slept, just across the road from my own rented room.

I return to this vignette to make a few further ingressions into the entangled domains of understanding, translation, and fieldwork. First, as implied above, Nani understood at least some of Jyoti's signing and crafted from her own understanding a "tellable" story (Labov 1972, cited in Savolainen 2017; Prasad 2010)—albeit one that was "impossible." Since putting-together may be the default mode through which people make sense of at least some natural sign utterances, this suggests that self-perceived understanding actually may contain, even obscure, misunderstanding and not-understanding. (This certainly includes my own.) Second, Nani was faced with a mismatch between what she understood Jyoti to have said—or what Nani put together such that she could tell a story—and what she understood about how the world works. She resolved this dissonance by assessing her tellable story of what Jyoti had said as impossible, rather than by reevaluating her own understanding, either of what Jyoti had said or of the world. In this sense her comments portrayed Jyoti as an intelligible narrator; you can only say someone has said something impossible if you have understood them, and if you have understood someone, they are by definition understandable, at least in that moment. Saying something impossible or untrue is thus evidence that you are intelligible. Yet to deem what Jyoti said "impossible" was also to portray her as an unreliable narrator—someone who might lie, not understand her own experiences, or say things that don't make sense. The crafting of a tellable story might be considered an act of care, and I consider it such; yet here the tellable story is also evaluated as impossible.

Third, this vignette and its analysis demonstrate that like Jyoti's neighbor, I too made, and continue to make, assumptions and evaluations that produce consequences. I assumed that Jyoti did not, in fact, sign to her neighbor that she and I had slept together; my analysis depends on my first-hand knowledge of an event that occurred but also on my assumption that the neighbor had understood incorrectly. And I told the neighbor what I thought had actually happened. Did my contradiction of the neighbor's interpretation of Jyoti's signing contribute to the neighbor thinking about and experiencing Jyoti as being difficult to understand? How might this be different than the neighbor thinking about her as saying "impossible" things? And here, in this text, I am keenly aware that my analysis positions Jyoti as failing to make sense to her neighbor and potentially as having a less complicated range of intentions than she no doubt had and has. That is to say, what if Jyoti wanted her neighbor to think that we had spent a night in the same home? At the same time, my analysis positions her neighbor as having failed in her own right. What I experience as acts motivated by the ethical demands of taking deaf signers seriously—acts of conversation and of analysis—have their own potential pitfalls.[5]

CAUGHT UP, CAUGHT IN, CAUGHT BY

On a warm June day in 2010, I sat chatting with Parvati and Shrila Khadka, deaf sisters-in-law, on their front porch. Parvati and Shrila lived in a house a fifteen-minute walk from the bazaar past forest and fruit trees. Their front porch faced a river valley and the green hills beyond it. Their gardens were lush with vegetables, and I loved when Shrila took me to look at them. Shrila's brother and mother— Parvati's husband and mother-in-law—had also been part of the household, but both had passed away before 2010. Parvati had three hearing sons, though the eldest was working abroad; his wife lived with the family. On that day in June, Sagar was filming us, and Parvati's second oldest son, Yug, was inside the house. As a participant and later as a repeated viewer of the video, I found our conversation frustrating and at times very painful, due in part to the content, as Parvati described someone hitting her, but also to my inability to fully understand. This scene does not yield a neat analysis or pithy conclusion but instead a chain of entangled questions and concepts, and I have included it to give a sense of the uncertainty of both conversation and analysis.[6]

Early in the video I ask Parvati some simple questions about her life in order to get us talking in front of the camera (lines 1–5 in the transcript in appendix 5). She tells me that her late husband had walked with a pronounced limp and that she had given birth to three sons (lines 6–8). Then Parvati launches into a story involving herself, Shrila, someone referred to as *JEṬHĀ* 'OLDEST,' a location downhill, and a man, perhaps associated with that location. Parvati also says that she was hit, and that a house fell apart (lines 10–16). In the moments between lines 16 and 17, Sagar and I briefly talk in NSL about the filming process; then the conversation between Parvati and me continues. I question her about what happened downhill, and Parvati says again that she was hit. Shrila tries to get my attention and emphasizes in both speech and sign that what happened was "over there." Parvati signs "GRAIN-ALCOHOL DRINK GRAIN-ALCOHOL DRINK HIT-self HIT-self" (line 22 part i) and then grabs Shrila and makes a shoving motion downward and to the side (line 22 part ii). The first part of her utterance unambiguously means that someone hit her. The directionality of the verb (Padden 1981), palm toward herself and hand moving inward, clearly indicates this; had she hit someone else, she would have turned her hand the other way and struck outward. There is, however, some ambiguity as to the phrase "GRAIN-ALCOHOL DRINK." GRAIN-ALCOHOL, as well as GRAIN-ALCOHOL DRINK, can refer to (drinking) alcohol, the effects of alcohol (drunkenness), or (a person from) a *jāt* 'caste/ ethnic group' typified as alcohol drinkers (Green 2022b).[7]

In the second part, when Parvati uses Shrila's body as a stand-in for another body, grabbing her and shoving her, it is less clear whether Parvati means "he grabbed and shoved me" or "I grabbed and shoved him." (It is also possible but less likely that Shrila's body represents Shrila herself; neither she nor Parvati indicated in any way that Shrila had been hurt during the narrated incident.) In line 25, I ask Parvati, "Point-Parvati MAN Point-Parvati?" and she confirms, yet it is not unambiguous what I was asking and therefore what she was answering. Literally, what I signed means something like "You(r) man?" Given pragmatic patterns, Parvati reasonably could have interpreted what I signed to mean "You're talking about a man?" or "This story is about you and a man?" or "Your man (i.e., your husband)?" In my next question I use the natural sign MARRIAGE, indicating that I am talking about her husband (line 27). Parvati responds quickly, "Point-self MAN WALKS-LIKE-THIS," moves her hand as if releasing or throwing something (a sign I cannot interpret in this context), signs "MAN" again, touches the porch on which she is sitting, and then signs "HOUSE, MAN *JEṬHĀ* 'OLDEST' Point-location HOUSE HIT HIT" (line 32). My best translation of this long utterance is: "My husband walked with a limp. [Utterance I don't know how to translate.] The oldest was here at the house. There was hitting."

The sign *JEṬHĀ* used in line 32 introduces additional ambiguity. Parvati regularly used this term to refer to both her husband, who was the oldest son in his family, and to her own oldest son; as discussed in chapter 3, birth-order terms are commonly used to refer to relatives, friends, and neighbors in both spoken Nepali and local sign. Concerned that Parvati was describing a scene of domestic violence, I ask, "Point-Parvati MAN *JEṬHĀ*?" and Parvati specifies that whether *jeṭhā* is husband or son, he is not the person who hit her: "Point-self *JEṬHĀ* HIT-self NEG 'my *jeṭhā* doesn't/didn't hit me'" (lines 33–34). Knowing that Parvati had talked in class before about being unhappy at home, I ask, "Does your second-oldest hit you?" Parvati again insists: "The person from downhill, the alcohol drinker/ person drinking alcohol, hit and shoved me!" (lines 37–38). Although she clearly separates her family members from the hitting, it remains unclear what the person referred to as *JEṬHĀ* is doing in this narrative. At this point Shrila takes a turn trying to explain the story to me, with Parvati chiming in (these turns are not in the appended transcript).

The video recording shows—and I remember—that I was able to follow and understand some parts of Parvati's story, but that I did not fully understand how the parts fit together. Who exactly had hit Parvati? What was the relationship between the hitting (lines 12, 14, 18, 22, 32, and 38) and the house falling apart (lines 16 and possibly 32)? How did "the oldest" fit in? I was troubled by Parvati's emotionally charged description of violence and wanted to understand more clearly. I also wanted to know whether someone more familiar with Parvati and her communication would understand what she was saying. I asked her son, Yug, to join us to help translate, and he agreed. With four of us now on camera, we settle onto the porch in a new configuration. I reinitiate conversation by asking Parvati about the alcohol-drinking person downhill (line 42). Parvati takes up the question immediately, and over the course of the next few turns (lines 43, 45, and 47) she repeats each of the elements raised in the initial narrative (lines 10–41), except for the alcohol drinker, whom I have just mentioned with Yug present and who is thus referentially present among this larger group of conversational participants. Parvati adds several more elements: the house was uphill, there was an earthquake, there were four relevant locations, and someone carried something on their back, and she directs a curse downhill with potent emotion.[8]

As Parvati finishes her turn, I direct my attention to Yug, tilting my head upward in a conventional questioning motion, but Yug shakes his head, laughing quietly (lines 48–49). Shrila at this point tries again to help us understand the story, pointing downhill and saying in Nepali "*yahā̃* 'here'" (pragmatically, "there") and several other words that I am unable to understand (line 50). Yug directs his question to his mother, though, asking in Nepali, "*ke bhayo* 'what happened?'" and using the conventional Q sign and corresponding questioning head movement (line 51). Parvati responds, again mentioning the earthquake and something falling apart, and adding a new detail: the height, and by conventional extension the age, of someone small and young (line 52). Yug again indicates that he hasn't understood (line 53).

Following Yug's second disavowal of understanding, I raise the topic of the man again, while Parvati simultaneously continues with her narrative, saying that she was pregnant with Yug (lines 54–55). "And the oldest male person?" I ask. "The oldest?" Parvati confirms. "The oldest male person," I repeat. To which Parvati replies with two signs: "EARTHQUAKE PUT-ON-BACK 'during the earthquake I put him on my back'" (lines 57–60). Sagar, Yug, and I each indicate that we have understood Parvati's most recent utterances: I respond with a nod (line 61) and in a mix of NSL and natural sign tell Sagar, who has sought my attention from off camera and presumably repeated what Parvati said, that yes, I understand she was pregnant with Yug (lines 61–63); and Yug begins to translate for the first time since I asked for his assistance. After making sure that I understand the Nepali words for earthquake, Yug explains, "*bhuichālā āũdākheri dājulāi bokhera lāgeko kahā̃ lānubhaera bhanuhunchha* 'She says when the earthquake came she picked up my older brother and carried him off [to safety]'" (lines 64–69).

As in the previous chapter, Yug's spoken translation serves both a referential function in its restatement of what has been said and a metalinguistic function in its rendering of sign as something that can be translated into speech (Jakobson 1959). Even though I was the only one who could fully hear what he had said, the fact of his speaking, and the expository facial expression that accompanied it—quite distinct from his expression of puzzlement—would most likely have also indicated to the deaf persons present that he had understood. At this point, his translation clearly accounted for some of the elements that Parvati had put into play: Parvati's and Jetha's presences, someone small and young (since Parvati's oldest son had been very young), someone carrying something (someone) on their back, and the earthquake itself. Indirectly, Yug's one-sentence story also accounted for Shrila's presence, as a member of the family, and for the house falling apart, as earthquakes destroy homes. It is also possible that one of the four locations was the house itself. The fact that Parvati was pregnant with Yug during the earthquake was not accounted for by Yug's translation, but it didn't need to be, as both Sagar and I had indicated our understanding of that element. In contrast, Yug's story did not account for Parvati getting hit, the alcohol drinker, the downhill location and/or person, and at least two remaining locations. Yet within the conversational unfolding, Yug's facial expression and translation had just marked Parvati as understood.

For better or worse, I wanted to know more and I kept asking questions. In other words, my determination to more fully understand Parvati inadvertently reintroduced the specter of not-understanding that had been socially if not referentially resolved in lines 61–69. In lines 70 and 71, I address Yug in spoken Nepali while Parvati continues her own train of thought, using Yug's physically present body as a stand-in for his physically absent older brother's much-younger narrativized body. I ask Parvati again about having been hit by a man, and she reiterates two elements: that this man was related to the downhill location and that he was a particular caste/ethnic group (lines 76–84). This time in addition to the local sign phrase GRAIN-ALCOHOL DRINK, she uses the NSL sign for a particular caste/ethnic group, which shows no resemblance to grain alcohol or drinking, thus resolving the prior ambiguity of the reference—or rather, resolving it in part, as she could have been indicating both that he was from a group typified as alcohol-drinking *and* that he was drinking or drunk. I ask, "And he hit you?" to which Parvati answers, "He hit me. My face was swollen like this" (lines 85–86). Yug watches her sign but ultimately concludes "*khoi thāhā bhaena*," literally, "Huh I don't know," or more idiomatically, "I have no idea" (line 87).

As in the previous chapter, when Binita said she did not understand Shrila, I wonder whether Yug "really" did not understand what his mother said in lines 84 and 86. Comparing the lines that Yug did translate (lines 58 and 60) with those he did not translate (84 and 86), the two sequences are very similar. *JEṬHĀ* (line 58) and GRAIN-ALCOHOL (line 84) are conventional signs, while PUT-ON-BACK (line 60) and SWOLLEN-LIKE-THIS (line 86) are immanent and transparent in context. The sign TO-HIT (line 86) is both conventional and immanent in the corporeal act of hitting. In lines 58 and 60 there is a setting (the earthquake), an object (the oldest son), and an action (put on back); the subject (Parvati) is implied. In lines 84 and 86 there is again an object (Parvati), an action (hit), and an implied subject (the man). In terms of a setting for the latter sequence, perhaps the location mentioned in line 77—downhill—could serve as one, although my sense is that it was meant more as a social identifier of the man—someone from downhill. More likely the earthquake or the period of time of the earthquake is the setting, given that in line 43, just after I asked about the man, Parvati's reply included the sign EARTHQUAKE, and the two stories were told together. Closely comparing the elements of these two sequences shows no obvious differences in terms of the conventionality and immanence or decipherability of signs nor in terms of information structure.

One option is that Yug robustly understood Parvati's story and decided not to translate. Perhaps he felt embarrassed or angry on behalf of himself or his mother. Another option is that he did not understand. My instinct is that the truth lies somewhere in between.[9] Despite the immanence of at least some of the signs Parvati produced, this is a more complicated situation than the one with Binita and Shrila. For one, Yug indicated that he understood Parvati at times; he translated the part of the story when Parvati talked about carrying his brother to safety, and he translated several other times during our filmed interactions that day, including a story about when his brother broke his arm while gathering fodder and a description of Parvati and her own brother as children. In addition, Yug was responding to a request from me for translation, which is a different cognitive and social (t)ask than being signed to with the expectation of a nontranslational response, as with Binita and Shrila.

My sense is that Yug understood individual elements of what Parvati had said, even when he did not translate—as did I. I can summarize in words the different moments what Parvati expressed something that Yug did not translate: she talked about being hit by a man downhill; told a story related to her natal home, perhaps involving cows; told another story about a relative in the police force and someone else, perhaps Parvati's mother-in-law; and discussed some relatives' family structure and place of residence. Whatever Yug was able to understand on a referential level of the unaccounted-for elements did not, it seems, make up a story that he experienced as or considered tellable—similar to how I have not been able to actually robustly *tell* the stories that I have just *mentioned*. Perhaps the story of how his mother picked up his brother during the earthquake was already familiar to Yug from previous tellings. Indeed, it is possible that not only his mother and aunt but also his hearing grandmother, who had only recently passed away, and other relatives had told it to him over and over in Nepali. In other words, perhaps what enabled Yug to translate the utterance in lines 58 and 60, "*JEṬHĀ* 'OLDEST'? EARTHQUAKE PUT-ON-BACK" was the connection of its referent to an event that Yug already knew about and that had already been rendered by others into a meaningful narrative.

I am not claiming that in natural sign, only already-known information can be communicated; many examples throughout the book make clear that such a claim would be insupportable. Indeed it is quite possible that Yug understood Parvati to say that a man had hit her (as did I, if not all the details), but did not want to say so, whether or not this was a story he had been told by her before. It is also possible that Yug understood bits and pieces—perhaps that there was a man and that someone was hit—but could not connect the parts to make a coherent story. Therefore I wonder if he had not already known the story about his mother carrying his brother, might he have understood the individual referents of her signs in lines 58 and 60 and yet been unable to figure out how they related to one another and thus translate them for me? The exigencies of emergent language, of tellability, of translation, and of what people feel comfortable saying in specific situations merge here in complex ways.

Moreover, understanding and translating begin to collapse into each other, in part due to my fieldwork practices. As suggested in chapter 4, interlocutors might understand and translate, understand and not translate, or not understand and not translate; this example indicates that someone might also partly understand and translate or partly understand and not translate. As discussed earlier, translating is a common practice within and across modalities in Maunabudhuk. However, requests for translation produce consequences, instigating implicit or explicit assessments of understanding and not-understanding. Yug did not provide a translation, and said aloud, "I don't know." And while understanding and not-understanding are definitionally in relation to the addressed person, *assessments* of understanding/not-understanding, including those conveyed by translations or their absences, accrue to the signer and their perceived intelligibility.

One could argue that understanding is not necessarily what is at stake in situations like these—that something else, like attention or time spent interacting together, is more important.[10] But the effort that Parvati put into repeating her story for us indicates that she wanted us to understand. Shrila too tried to help Yug and me understand. In fact, her input raises a serious question about how to analyze local signing practices as well as translation. She seemed to understand Parvati's story: if not every specific utterance Parvati made, then at least the event to which she was referring. Yet what Shrila said did not enable me to grasp the story, and Yug focused only on his mother. Jakobson (1959:261) writes that for both "linguists and . . . ordinary word-users, the meaning of any linguistic sign is its translation into some further, alternative sign," whether through rewording (into the same language), translation proper (into another language), or transmutation (into a nonlinguistic semiotic system).[11]

Was Shrila rewording (translating within a language) or was she responding with further comments or elaboration? Either way, the story felt caught—caught not so much in natural sign, as in the minds of Parvati and Shrila, as well as in the space between them. It is this conversation that I think of when arguing Saussure's model of the talking head should not be dismissed. As per the introduction, in this model, Person A thinks something and voices it; upon hearing what Person A says, what Person A thought appears in Person B's mind. Understanding is achieved! Obviously, the model does not account for people who communicate through sign, tactile language, or writing. But that is not generally the criticism people level at Saussure; rather they focus on the model's simplicity. And as this chapter shows, it is overly simple; understanding is a multilayered, ongoing dance of multiple processes, simultaneously cognitive and corporeal, interactional and ethical. Yet the model also captures something real; and that realness becomes especially clear, and painful, when it fails. I could not get into my own mind what Parvati, and Shrila, had in theirs and deeply, urgently wanted to convey to me, wanted me to understand.

UNRELIABILITY, LIES, AND GRAMMAR

In mid-September I encountered Jyoti carrying a load of firewood, one of the jobs she did for pay and meals. She had a swollen eye and told me that her brother and sister-in-law had been yelling at her. I asked her about her swollen eye. At first I thought she was saying someone had hit her, but through further questions and her responses, I understood that she had gotten hurt while cutting firewood. And, as I wrote in my fieldnotes, some hearing people present "elaborated for me when I asked her in front of [them], and they explained that the wood itself had hit her." The following morning Krishna Gajmer and Sagar, who had been talking with Jyoti while drinking tea before class, said that Jyoti had attributed her swollen eye to a hornet or wasp sting, though when I asked her she repeated that a piece of wood had bounced up and struck her eye. Both Sagar and Krishna appeared frustrated, and Sagar said that the particular quality of the swelling looked like it had been caused by a bite not a blow.[12]

While in this case neither Sagar nor Krishna directly accused Jyoti of lying, I did observe people explicitly say that a signer had lied. In late October I ran into Parvati's middle son's best friend while out walking. I asked if Parvati had gone to her *māitighar* 'natal home' for Dasai, a holiday that fell during mid-October in 2010, and he said yes. We talked about how long she had stayed there during her last visit at Tij, a holiday that fell during mid-September in 2010. He said that she had only been there a couple days, and I said no, it was much longer than that, around two weeks. When I said this, he replied, "*malāi ḍā̃ṭnubhayo* 'she lied to me.'" I offered, "Maybe she meant two weeks," but he said, "No, she said two days." He showed what she had said, holding up two fingers, and I again suggested that perhaps she had meant two weeks. Later, when writing down fieldnotes, however, I realized that Parvati never expressed time in terms of weeks (nor did any local signers so far as I saw). It occurred to me that perhaps she was not lying so much as answering a different question, one that she had understood but that he hadn't asked.[13]

It is easy to imagine how such a conversation would have proceeded. He might have pointed to her natal village and then formed the Q sign, meaning, "How long were you there?" She might easily—and not incorrectly—have interpreted his question to mean something like "Tell me about your trip." Perhaps her reported reply, "Two," meant, in her internal script, something like "My sister-in-law and I both went." But he, following the ongoing script in his head, assumed she meant "I was there for two days." The plausibility of this imagined scenario is supported by the exchange between Krishna's older brother Samman and Sagar, described in chapter 3, during which Samman asked Sagar where he lived, but Sagar thought he was asking if his home was similar to Samman's and Krishna's. When utterances are lean, it seems, people may elaborate them mentally in different ways, leading to miscommunication.

What strikes me about my conversation with Parvati's son's best friend is that he did not assume that he might have misunderstood Parvati, that she might have misunderstood him, or for that matter that I might be wrong or lying. Instead, he assumed she was purposefully misleading him and telling him things that were not true. Fricker (2017) might call this an instance of "epistemic injustice," which Kidd, Medina, and Pohlhaus Jr. (2017:1) define as "forms of unfair treatment that relate to issues of knowledge, understanding, and participation in communicative practices." Parvati's son's best friend was not the only one who assumed that she lied, and Parvati was not the only person who was disbelieved. Several people told me directly that both Parvati's and Shrila's claims that a relative hit them should not be believed. Jyoti's claim that her younger brother hit her was also disputed. In one case a woman in the bazaar responded to Shrila by telling her to "hit . . . back." I asked if she believed what Shrila said, and the woman said, "No, not at all, it's just what she says," so she gives her a reply. On another occasion, Parvati made the same complaint, and a hearing man angrily signed "*CHHIḤ* 'TO-HECK-WITH-YOU" at her and then told her, in speech, to stop telling lies. The other hearing men gathered nearby agreed that she was lying. However, a worker at the health post told me that they were not treated well by their family.[14]

There are several possibilities here. One very real possibility is that they were telling the truth. Violence among people who live together is well-documented, and people who are multiply marginalized, such as deaf and disabled women, may experience heightened levels of violence.[15] In this case families and neighbors doubting their stories inflicts additional emotional violence and leaves them with little social recourse. I do want to note, however, that Jyoti frequently spent time away from her home, demonstrating agency over her body and movement. It is also possible that some or all of Shrila's, Parvati's, and Jyoti's claims were lies or exaggerations; to state otherwise would deny that deaf natural signers can inhabit the same range of subject positions and communicative stances that NSL signers and hearing speakers can. A third, not-mutually-exclusive possibility is this: What if these women's relatives had *threatened* to hit them or had raised a hand *as if* threatening to hit them, as a way of indicating anger, and what if the signers were referring to such an instance but were understood as describing a completed action? Related to this possibility, what if certain actions metonymically represent emotional states, but not all addressees recognize this?

One day, Parvati told me that she had cried when her son, Yug, returned to his job abroad. Her daughter-in-law (Yug's sister-in-law) said that no one had cried. Assuming that Parvati was not referring to having cried in private, perhaps she used the sign CRY to describe her emotions; perhaps CRY can also mean "sad" or "anguished." Similarly, perhaps HIT also means "angry." Signs for physical confrontation did sometimes seem to stand in for verbal confrontations. For example, when Bal Limbu complained that his employer did not pay him properly, Sanu Kumari Limbu told Bal that he should refuse to work and that he was being cheated because he's deaf. Krishna chimed in that Sanu Kumari should go tell the owner that herself, and imitated rolling up his sleeves for a confrontation. I do not think that he was actually suggesting that Sanu Kumari, an elderly woman, was going to physically tussle with Bal's employer, though he could have been suggesting an imagined fight humorously.[16]

And even if signs like CRY and HIT do not conventionally—for particular signers or across signers—mean anything other than "cry" and "hit," perhaps Parvati, Shrila, and Jyoti were using the available signs to express profound dissatisfaction with their lives; perhaps they were doing their best to say that they felt abused, mistreated, or sad, even if they had not literally cried or been hit—and again, I am not claiming that they were not but instead trying to think about the entanglement of accusations and disbelief with natural sign as a communicative practice. With these examples, along with instances when Sagar or I, or both of us, guessed what someone had meant incorrectly or at least incompatibly with each other, I noticed a pattern.[17]

Many instances of misunderstanding involve two linguistic domains: mood and action-based metaphors. By mood, I mean the grammatical encoding of the relationship of an action (e.g., hitting something) to reality. That is to say, actions do not only or merely occur. They may be what in English I can describe as threatened, portended, possible, impossible, likely, unlikely, desired, feared, or about to happen; the exact articulation of these kinds of relationships is language-specific. By action-based metaphors, I mean the rhetorical mention of an action to stand not for itself but for something related to it—for example, hitting for anger, or crying for sadness. While metaphor and mood are seldom discussed together in linguistics (Taverniers 2006 is an exception), the two are united in that in each case a reported action may or may not have actually happened (where "actually" is relative; in this framework a kiss between fictional characters in a story would be actual—so long as within the narrative, it happened between them and not in a daydream).

Returning to another vignette from chapter 3, recall that one morning in May 2010, Jyoti and I had a conversation about how her sister-in-law had drunkenly spilled water on the previous afternoon. Following our conversation, Jyoti and I entered the NSL classroom where Sagar told me that the day prior she had said something to him about a fight, or about slapping someone or getting slapped. He wondered if she was "tricking" him. I relayed the story she had just told me, and then asked Jyoti directly about whether slapping had been involved. I understood her to reply that she had rolled up her sleeves, threatening to hit her sister-in-law for being drunk while carrying water.[18]

What if Jyoti had, on the previous day, described to Sagar her reaction to her sister-in-law's drunken mishaps, and Sagar had interpreted her as narrating an actual event, while Jyoti had depicted herself as being angry, threatening her sister-in-law, or perhaps wanting to hit her, whether in the moment or when telling the story? Another instance supports this interpretation, and emphasizes that I was as likely as anyone else to misunderstand (here, unsurprisingly, in the process of trying to establish further certainty). On the morning of October 1, Jyoti repeatedly talked about her sister-in-law getting her wrists and ankles tied together and hauled off to jail by the police. Although I intuited that she meant that she wanted this to happen, or predicted that it would happen, I nevertheless tried to find out if perhaps it had happened, by asking (or trying to ask), "Did this already happen? Is your *buhāri* 'sister-in-law' at home?" It is difficult to say whether I actually communicated these meanings with my utterances, but I interpreted her answers—an affirmative to the first and negative to the second—in relation to what I knew I wanted to say (i.e., to my internal script of our ongoing conversation). Jyoti then went to talk to Uma Didi, the owner of the tea shop where we all frequently ate, who told me that Jyoti "was saying that she was telling her *buhāri* that she'd get hauled off to jail."[19]

In the hitting case, the distinction between a threat or desire and an occurrence caused confusion. In the arresting case, the distinction between a prediction or warning and an occurrence caused confusion. Other instances of possible misunderstanding, recorded in my fieldnotes or inscribed in my memory, center on similar distinctions. I remember, for example, multiple times when Shrila told Sagar and me that her daughter-in-law had thrown Shrila's notebook in the toilet and then showed up the following day with said notebook. I wonder if the daughter-in-law had actually threatened to throw the notebook away (e.g., by holding the notebook near the toilet) or had signed that she would throw it away (e.g., by pointing to the toilet and to the notebook and making a throwing sign), and if in fact Shrila was actually telling us that and we misinterpreted her. Similarly, Sagar and I once understood Parvati to be claiming that a relative was pregnant by a man who was not her husband. Later she criticized the woman's inappropriate behaviors without mentioning the pregnancy.[20] In retrospect, I wonder whether Parvati was telling us that the relative could get pregnant, that she was worried about such an eventuality, or perhaps that she had told her relative that she could get pregnant.

On a different occasion, Padma Puri, Krishna, Sagar, and I had a conversation about cross-caste practices revolving around the acceptance or refusal by dominant ("high" or *ṭhulo* 'large') castes of food and water from members of marginalized ("low," "untouchable," or *sāno* 'small') castes. The topic came up because we were talking about going to Padma's later that day, and Krishna said that Sagar and I had come to his house. Padma asked if we had eaten there and I said no but that we had had water. Padma seemed somewhat surprised that I would accept water from Krishna or at Krishna's home. I asked if Padma would accept food and water from Krishna (question 1). At first I thought that he answered no, and Sagar seemed to think that as well, because he reminded Padma of his Maoist sensibilities. (While at that time none of the major political parties were advocating for relegalizing caste discrimination, the Maoists were the biggest party most explicitly fighting against ongoing caste- and ethnicity-based oppression.) Padma then pointed out that at the tea shop, he willingly drinks water that Krishna pours for him. I wondered "aloud" in sign if maybe the rules were different at someone's home, and asked again if Padma would eat if Krishna cooked him food and offered it to him (question 2).[21]

This time Padma said yes. At the time of the conversation, I thought he was changing his mind, but that evening when I recorded the conversation in my field-notes, another possibility occurred to me. In asking Padma if he would accept food from Krishna, I probably signed something like "Point-Krishna COOK EAT DRINK?" with a questioning head tilt during the articulation of EAT and DRINK. Critically, this utterance could also be used to ask about past events. Thus, while I meant "Would you accept food from Krishna?," Padma may well have understood me to mean "Have you accepted food from Krishna?" In the language of this chapter, the scripts we were following in the first instance may have diverged in our minds without doing so in our signs. The second time I asked the question, it seems that we were both in the hypothetical mode.[22]

There are several ways to account for these domains of increased potential misunderstanding. I could claim that:

1. Natural sign as used in Maunabudhuk and Bodhe does not have grammatical or pragmatic conventions to express certain moods or to distinguish between action as description versus action as metaphor.
2. These grammatical or pragmatic conventions do exist, but only some signers use them.
3. These grammatical or pragmatic conventions do exist, but only some addressees understand them.

In fact I did see signers differentiate between HIT and RAISE-ONE'S-HAND, although it could be unclear if the latter meant "to be about to hit" or "to raise one's hand as if about to hit but only to express anger." And if conventions exist, but not everyone uses them (and those people who do not, don't have a different convention), what kind of conventionality is that—or rather, what to make of an uneven distribution of conventions, both among deaf people and across deaf and hearing people? How might I differentiate among natural sign, its usage, and its users, and what are the analytic and ethical stakes of different means of doing so?

If some signers and not others command certain forms or expressions, do I say that some are less competent than others? To do so seems highly problematic given that signers never seemed to be in doubt about what they themselves were saying. Or should I say that there are as many sets of conventions as there are signers and that different sets have different features? While this option is tempting, it dismisses conventions across signers and the ways in which those conventions matter for communication. It also displaces questions of difference from actual practices to abstract systems, a move that could be generative in its focus on form yet incomplete in its erasure of context-specific use. And where in this are addressees? If natural sign scaffolds on nonlinguistic knowledge, and if addressees must put together parts of utterances, then would it not be the *addressees'* conventions and competences on which I should focus my attention? Yet even if I do so, when *no* addressee can understand, or when, as in the case of the extended example with Parvati and Shrila, another deaf local signer understands but understanding is not achieved between deaf local signers and others, the locus of not-understanding does not feel like it matters nearly so much as the not-understanding itself.

SUSPICION

Another way of thinking about issues of understanding and misunderstanding was suggested by Tok Bahadur Pradhan, a hearing man who in 2010 had been teaching deaf students for sixteen years. In late September 2010, Sagar, who was his former student, and I went to visit him at the deaf school in Mulghat, and then Tok returned with us to Maunabudhuk to talk to the parents of several deaf children about sending their kids to school. He also sat in on the NSL class, where Shrila upon meeting him immediately said, "My *buhāri* 'daughter-in-law' yells at me, come talk to her [on my behalf]." He did. Without accusing the younger hearing woman of yelling or mistreating the older deaf women, he said that deaf people are often very suspicious, because they so often miss what's going on around them. Therefore, he said, it is important to be especially clear about what one is doing; for example, if you ask them not to eat some sweets, tell them that no one is allowed to eat the sweets.[23]

While cautious about a generalization as broad as "deaf people are suspicious," I nevertheless want to take seriously what Tok Bahadur said. I did not record the Nepali word that Tok Bahadur used, but I want to be clear that I use the word *suspicion* here descriptively: to characterize how people may encounter the world and other people in that world as unjust, deceitful, or withholding of information. In Maunabudhuk and Bodhe, deaf people—even the ones whose families most actively communicate with them—are so frequently in situations where hearing people speak and do not translate what they say into sign. In spaces where there were deaf people present, I witnessed spoken, untranslated discussions about bus schedules, casual conversations about what the children in the family were up to that day, news about a neighboring family, and reminiscences about working in the Gulf States. I have no evidence that these kinds of things *can't* be said in local sign—on the contrary—but frequently they *aren't*.[24]

Deaf signers may be able to understand spoken interaction to varying degrees, including by tracking bodily movements and postures and their integration with visible activities. For example, Sagar once informed me that Sanu Kumari was telling me something in speech about tomorrow; he had inferred this from a particular forward thrust of the chin.[25] But when speech carries the majority of referential content, deaf signers are made to miss a great deal (De Meulder et al. 2019). Deaf people who lip-read also point out the labor entailed in doing so and the impossibility of getting everything (e.g., Kolb 2013). Kushalnagar et al. (2020) describe this kind of failure to ensure that deaf family members are able to access conversations around them as a form of communicative neglect. In the context of DeafBlind signers in the United States, Edwards (2014: 107–108) describes the frustration of a DeafBlind woman who would put her hands on signers to perceive their conversation—and the signers would "freeze." Using Goffman's (1981) framework, being an overhearer and/or a ratified but unaddressed recipient is as important a participant role as speaker/signer and addressee.

I understand Tok Bahadur to have been saying that deaf people are suspicious because hearing people frequently say things in speech without signing, and therefore deaf people may not have the same perspective on events that they would if they had been able to see to what had been said—or, to invoke NSL signers, if the hearing people had bothered to sign with and around them. Using Tok Bahadur's example of sweets, a deaf person told directly, "Don't eat that," might not know that everyone else was told the same thing, or that the plan—said aloud but not signed—was for everyone to eat the sweets together that evening. In this scenario there are two key propositions: first, that the deaf person in question has not actually been mistreated but only thinks they have been; and second, that their assumptions nevertheless make sense because of asymmetrical access to information. Interestingly, when spending time in deaf society, I found that deaf NSL signers themselves are sometimes skeptical of natural signers' tales of hardships.[26] NSL signers also frequently report that they have been lied to or cheated by hearing people. Hearing people absolutely take advantage of and mistreat deaf people (and other hearing people). I am also familiar with cases where, at least from my perspective, more robust mutual understanding on a referential level might have changed both parties' perspectives. Although Tok Bahadur did not say so, hearing people are also frequently skeptical about what signers say, or what they think signers say, as this chapter shows.

In considering hearing people's skepticism toward deaf signers and deaf people's skepticism toward hearing people and sometimes other deaf people, both in

Maunabudhuk and beyond, I want to take seriously the possibility that frequent misunderstandings are fertile ground for the cultivation of an epistemological stance of suspicion. In the case of deaf people, suspicion can be one possible consequence of communicative neglect, and in the case of both deaf and hearing people, of repeated misunderstandings. Anthropologists have similarly documented how rumors flourish in particular settings and environments (e.g., Das 2007). I want to state again that I am not claiming that Jyoti's, Parvati's, and Shrila's complaints were untrue or based on misunderstandings or on missed information that if they had had access to would have prompted them to feel and experience things differently. Nevertheless, Tok Bahadur's point that deaf people may very reasonably encounter the world with suspicion is worth considering, especially in concert with NSL signers' insistence that it is within hearing people's capacities to communicate with deaf people, and yet hearing people often choose not to.

CONCLUSION

It might be argued that the kinds of communicative situations described in this chapter are widely familiar; all modes of communication involve the potential for partial understanding, misunderstanding, gaps, accusations, and dismissals. What is particular about natural signers? It is helpful to return again to the experiences of Nepali Sign Language signers. NSL signers sometimes easily interact with hearing people who do not know NSL, using natural sign and/or resources from spoken or written language, but they are not strangers to finding themselves made unintelligible by hearing people. And natural signers sometimes communicate easefully with hearing people. Critically, however, the experiences of NSL signers and (some) natural signers have different temporal and social horizons. For an NSL user a moment or even repeated moments of frustrated, frustrating, or failed communication with hearing people contrast with a remembered past and anticipated future of intelligible interactions with other NSL signers. For (some) natural signers, however, the juxtaposition between making sense and not making sense is typical; there is no other way. Put differently, the unpredictable ubiquity of both intelligible and unintelligible interactions is not just *a* norm—as it can be for NSL signers as well in their interactions outside of deaf society—it is for (some) natural signers *the* norm.

When analyzing statements that get socially evaluated as to truthfulness—whether they concern drinking and eating, relationships with kin, violence, or affection—there are various possible approaches. From one perspective the truth-value may not matter; what matters more is that they are utterances with affective meaning beyond referential facticity. From another perspective the truth-value very much matters, because its evaluation has social consequences; that is to say, when people frequently disbelieve other people, the fabric of sociality is affected. These options might be applied in any situation where people are thought to have lied. I am haunted, however, by the degree to which, in Maunabudhuk, for these particular signers, questions of truth are inextricably entangled in the social and semiotic limits and possibilities of the communicative mode.

Through a series of conversations among deaf residents of Maunabudhuk and Bodhe, their hearing families, Sagar, and me, I have also considered whether at times my insistence on a certain kind of understanding rendered people more vulnerable to being regarded as unintelligible. Several times hearing signers told me a deaf signer was lying, when I thought the former had misunderstood the latter. In one sense, calling someone a liar in these circumstances entrenches them in a kind of nonintelligibility, yet in another sense, assuming that one has understood properly, even if what one has understood is a lie, is definitionally assuming that the other is understandable. Conversely, by assuming that deaf people are not (necessarily) lying, I have also had to assume that hearing people have not properly made sense of deaf signers—which as I argued in chapter 1 definitionally means that the signers did not make sense to their addressees. Sagar was frequently far more suspicious of local signers' stories (especially those that involved complaints or violence), sometimes asking me if they were lying or tricking him. And yet by asking this question, he also assumed that sense-making had occurred.

For the most part, the people whom I found the hardest to understand were also generally treated by their co-residents as people who lied, were not "with it" or worth engaging in conversation, or of whom might one say *"ke bhanchha, bhanchha."* Jyoti, Parvati, and Shrila were generally evaluated as making less sense, being more likely to lie, and so forth than the other natural signers with whom I worked closely in these villages. While recognizing that I do not and cannot know these women's histories or subjective experiences, I keep coming back to this: intelligibility requires a presumption of intelligibility for it to be achieved interactively; thus the absence of such a presumption perpetuates unintelligibility. Are people hard to understand because they are hard to understand or because (since they are [assumed to be] hard to understand) others have not tried very hard to understand them? What, over time, does a failure to be attended to, responded to fully or in part, believed, engaged with, understood, or taken seriously, produce in a person's communicative and social habits and practices? How does getting treated over and over as if you make no sense seep into your very bones?

Moreover, negative evaluations, which I think of as the residue of iterative miscommunications, accrue not only to specific people but also more generally to the fact of being deaf and communicating in sign. Even the most communicatively adept and socially respected deaf persons are not unfailingly understood, and negative assumptions about particular people leak into broader understandings of what it is to be deaf or a signer. In the summer of 2012, I returned to Maunabudhuk, almost two years after I had last been there. I spent my first night in the bazaar with plans to visit the hamlets where most of my deaf friends and acquaintances lived in the following days. Although my hearing friends and acquaintances in the bazaar all immediately recognized me, several hearing people expressed doubt that the deaf people—with whom I had spent even more time—would remember me. I sensed that this potential forgetfulness was being attributed to some quality of deaf persons or deafness. One of the hearing people later named this association directly. Plying me with hot tea and freshly fried snacks, she wondered aloud if the deaf people would remember me, then moved her hands in the air as if signing and said, "*hāt chalāūdāi* 'they move their hands [like this].'"[27]

In doing so, she located the source of their projected forgetfulness in signing, the communicative modality characteristic of deaf people. She did not identify any particular deaf people, and it is unclear to me if she was thinking specifically about the women focused on in this chapter—that is to say, the women who lived closest to the bazaar and who therefore were most likely to regularly interact with bazaar residents. But why would deaf people, including these particular deaf people, have forgotten me? While these women were more likely to encounter communicative difficulties than hearing people, and than many other local signers, none of them experienced memory loss or had trouble recognizing faces. So why were other residents wondering if they would know who I was?

Here I harken back to the figure of the deaf or *lāṭo* person as discussed in chapter 1 and to the kinds of assumptions and expectations sutured to it. If being made *lāṭo* is a relational process, it is critical to name the elements involved. I have argued that grammar does ethical labor, and that in natural sign, less elaborated, less conventional, and less shared grammar means that people have to do more work than in conventional languages. In other words, the relational process of (un)intelligibility includes both the communicative material and its speakers/signers and addressees. The lean quality of natural sign is both a constraint and an affordance, in that it leaves room for people to engage in sense-making—and room for them to choose to do so or not. Moreover, the consequences of those choices are not bound to specific interactional moments but extend beyond them into the broader fabric of communicative sociality between and among deaf and hearing signers.

Perhaps it is unnecessary to do so, but I nevertheless note here that not a single deaf person failed to know exactly who I was.

Afterword

Across the introduction and five chapters, this book has made a series of inter-woven interventions. Chapter 1 centered deaf NSL signers' insights as valuable both empirically and theoretically and documented how NSL signers objectify, name, and characterize natural sign—as a mode of signed communication that has expansive possibilities but also limits. NSL signers' discourse further reveals that communicative vulnerability can—and should—be located in participant configurations, not individuals, and that natural sign conversations are especially vulnerable to the whims of hearing participants. Drawing on NSL signers' perspectives, this book argues that natural sign is a phenomenon in the world, and one that offers particular purchase on the entanglement of language, interaction, and ethics. It shows that language is not only a medium for ethical engagement but also and more foundationally its result.

I have also argued that understanding natural sign requires attending to its particular sociolinguistic and semiotic features. A common idea in sign language studies is that of the critical mass: the number of deaf people necessary for the emergence of a signed language (e.g., Kegl, Senghas, and Coppola 1999), whether in a school or a community such as a village. Numbers are not all that matter; how often people communicate, whether they know each other well, and what kinds of shared backgrounds can be assumed also affect the process and structure of language (Meir et al. 2010; Padden 2011). Sign language scholars interested in the relationship between communities of signers and sign itself often formulate their analyses in relation to forms and features, particular dimensions of linguistic structure, and demographics. I have suggested that underneath these more technical-seeming issues are existential questions about who understands whom, who gets to take language for granted, and who does not. Do people want to communicate with each other? What other communicative and other demands are being made on them? What kinds of assumptions of intelligibility are overtly and implicitly made? How do deaf and hearing people understand each other, as well as misunderstand and not-understand, and how do they evaluate their interactions? Put another way, language emergence is not only a demographic issue, it is also an ethical one.

In chapter 2, I explored the particular demographics of natural sign in Maunabudhuk and Bodhe, arguing that there is evidence of transmission across time (and space), and yet that it is not an emerging sign language. Analyzing deaf demography in Maunabudhuk and Bodhe, I showed that the simultaneous possibilities and precarities of natural sign are linked to the fact that it is widely available and used, but not the primary communicative mode for a dense or tightly connected social group. My analysis lead me to argue that deaf people's presence in the world is much less exceptional than is often implied, and the world far more sign-saturated.

In chapter 3, I theorized natural sign's constraints and affordances in relation to conventionality, immanence, and emergence. I demonstrated how the fact that natural sign does not interpellate its addressees the way conventional grammar does creates time and space in which people may or may not do the work—as NSL signers know. Whether or not people make sense of natural sign depends in many cases on their willingness to do so. In chapters 4 and 5, I offered accounts of interactions within specific contexts. In doing so, I showed how deaf and hearing interlocutors' orientations toward communicating in natural sign has effects on that communication and in turn how repeated difficulties in communication affect people's desires, expectations, and practices. Deaf natural signers creatively shape, and are also shaped by, their communicative circumstances, both in particular interactions and over the course of their lives.

These arguments matter intellectually and they matter socially and politically. Founding assumptions in social and linguistic theory, but also in social life, appear differently when theorized from the perspective of users of signed (and) emergent language. Signed language, whether emergent or not, demands much closer attention to perception, to senses, and to access than scholars outside of sign language studies, deaf studies, and "deaf anthropology" (Friedner and Kusters 2020) often offer—and as I argue in the introduction, *all* language use, even in hypothetical situations, should garner such attention, so as not to naturalize some bodies and erase others. Emergent language in turn demands attention to attention, along with attention to intention, care, apathy, desire, refusal, ethics, and the ways that the boundary between language and everything else is both sharp and porous.

This book does not claim that if only people would try, they would always understand each other across sensory, linguistic, and other differences. Sometimes people try and fail. Sometimes people have other labor they need to do: caring for children, earning a living. What this book does claim, and demonstrate, is that even in the absence of the resources of conventional language that most people in the world take for granted, people can draw on linguistic conventions, however lean, social and corporeal knowledge and routines, and a shared desire to communicate, to take up the world's nudges, wrest immanent signs into actuality, and work to understand each other. The existence of natural sign, the ways people communicate in it, and the observations NSL signers make together suggest that deaf-centered sociality and access to conventional signed languages are critical for deaf children and adults. Yet these same things also suggest that communication among deaf people and between deaf and hearing people that does not involve conventional language, that makes use of other available resources, can and does produce connection, communication, and communicative sociality.[1] While different from shared sign languages and deaf community sign languages, natural sign makes communication among deaf people, and between deaf and hearing people, eminently possible. And to return to the tensions described in the introduction, natural signers' communicative vulnerability also demands acknowledgment, as is so powerfully laid out by NSL signers' discourse.

Translation is also a key theme across multiple of these chapters. It is present in a variety of contexts: in conversations within natural sign or NSL, between natural sign and NSL, between signing and speaking, and among signing, speaking, and writing. As the final chapter shows, translating can transform something that is partially understood into something that is socially rendered as fully understood, misunderstood, or not understood at all. Even with the best translations, translating is a complicated endeavor; in the contexts written about here, translation can render a person both intelligible (you have been understood well enough to be translated) and unintelligible (you are a person who requires translation). I have sometimes thought of translation, especially of lean utterances into more elaborated ones, as an act of love, care, or responsibility. But love itself is complicated and fraught. Love can overstep. Love, like translation, can get things wrong, misdirect, change things in unintended ways. I am thinking here of how NSL signers would frequently facilitate conversations with NEW NSL signers whom I had just met, translating and often adding to what had been said. At times I found this mediation helpful, even necessary. Other times I found myself asking them to let the other person and I communicate directly, together, even if we struggled. My instinct is that my conversational partners also experienced translations and augmentations as sometimes relieving and other times frustrating.

In certain respects, then, this book is about translation; and it is also a practice of translation. Translation is present in the literal translations I have made from natural sign, NSL, and Nepali to English, and in the more figurative translations I have made from fieldwork experiences to ethnographic text, from countless hours of interactions to the pages you are reading. While these translations have been for me an act of love, I recognize the ambivalence of love, the ways I have undoubtedly misunderstood and not-understood. And (but?) there are forms of love and relationality that sidestep translation altogether. Once again, I turn to my interlocutors to make sense.

On May 24, 2010, I recorded in my fieldnotes an interaction between Parvati Kadgha and myself into which I drew Padma Puri and Sagar Karki, asking them to help me understand what she had said. Parvati was telling me about a *pujā* 'ceremony, ritual'; she also mentioned her sons. Sagar and Padma were able to understand more than I had, explaining to me that the *pujā* involved ghee and a sacrificial goat, though neither of them was able to pinpoint exactly who would be there and when it would happen. Padma described for me in detail how the goat's throat was cut, and then its blood spread and its head offered up, and said that the temple in question was located in the Tarai, the plains to our south. Sagar turned his attention back to Parvati, teasing her about the ghee. He depicted her waiting until no one else was around, then opening a bottle of the rich food and scooping handfuls into her mouth, all the while keeping watch to make sure no one was coming. Parvati, along with everyone else, laughed at the scene he created. Unsurprisingly, I wanted to know who, when, why, and for how long.

None of us, in other words, seemed to fully understand what Parvati was telling us. While I indicated directly that I had not understood, Sagar and Padma were more equivocal. Neither of them translated or reworded what she had said, nor did they say that they could not do so. Instead, each of them took up a thread from her signing and wove it into something new. Padma responded by sharing his own knowledge and experiences, while Sagar focused on one dimension of the story that he had fully understood—the ghee—and created a different kind of communicative event, teasing Parvati in a recognizable, socially appropriate way. Both Padma and Sagar's actions indicated that they had, at least in part, understood her. By expanding on what Parvati had signed, and in Sagar's case directly addressing her, they rendered her at that moment intelligible as a signer, a participant in multiparty conversation and communicative sociality. Whether or not they fully made sense of what she said, they made her into someone who made sense.

Deaf Population in Maunabudhuk and Bodhe

TABLE A.1 Calculating the deaf population in Maunabudhuk and Bodhe

	Lowest number of deaf people	Highest number of deaf people	Lowest total population	Highest total population	Lowest percentage deaf (%)	Highest percentage deaf (%)
Maunabudhuk	24	29	2,569	2,966	0.8	1.1
Bodhe	19	48	3,056	3,056	0.6	1.6

SOURCE: Green (2014c:79) details the provenance of these numbers.

Signing and Sign Communities: English-Language Categories and Logics

SOCIOSPATIAL CATEGORIES

TABLE A.2 Primary sociospatial categories

Name of type of signing and associated community of signers	Stated or implied characteristics of signing	Stated or implied characteristics of community of signers	Examples
• Deaf community sign language, national sign language (overlapping categories) • Deaf or deaf community	• Conventional language with properties like compositionality, paradigmatic opposition, etc. • For national sign languages, used in parts or all of a country or across more than one country	• Presence of educational institutions, deaf-run organizations • Most signers are deaf	American Sign Language Idioma de Señas de Nicaragua Israeli Sign Language Kenyan Sign Language Nepali Sign Language
• Shared sign language, village sign language (often but not always used synonymously) • Shared signing community, deaf village	• Conventional language • Frequently has linguistic features that differ from deaf community sign languages	• High incidence of (genetic) deafness, at least several generations deep • Often rural setting • Deaf and hearing signers	Adamorobe Sign Language Al-Sayyid Bedouin Sign Language Ban Khor Sign Language Kata Kolok

TABLE A.2 Continued

Name of type of signing and associated community of signers	Stated or implied characteristics of signing	Stated or implied characteristics of community of signers	Examples
• Home sign • Home signer	• Somewhat to highly systematic	• Classically described as initiated by one deaf person who does not learn a previously existing language • Hearing family members participate to varying degrees	David's home sign (US) *Mímicas* (Nicaragua)

A FULLER LIST OF SOCIOSPATIAL CATEGORIES

alternate sign language

CULTURE

deaf community sign language

family sign

family sign language

home sign

- communal homesign
- family homesign
- individual homesign systems
- oral home sign
- multigenerational homesign
- rural home sign
- shared homesign systems

indigenous sign language

institutionalized sign language

local sign(s)

local sign language

macrocommunity

making hands

microcommunity

national sign language

natural sign

nucleated sign networks

original sign language

regional sign language

rural sign language

shared sign language

spontaneous sign

urban sign language

village sign language

Note: The term "indigenous sign language" has sometimes been used as a near-synonym for "village sign language," but Fox Tree (2011) argues that conflating them erases the specificity of indigeneity as a social category.

TEMPORAL CATEGORIES

TABLE A.3 Primary temporal categories

Name of type of signing	Stated or implied characteristics of signing	Examples
• Emerging sign languages (community type varies)	• Younger than established sign languages • Emergence within a few cohorts/generations • Rapidly changing	Al-Sayyid Bedouin Sign Language Israeli Sign Language
• Established sign languages (community type varies)	• Older than emerging sign languages • Changing less rapidly than emerging sign languages	Adamorobe Sign Language American Sign Language

Hou and de Vos (2022:118) also note the use of terms like "new, young, first/second generation, conventional, mature . . . or institutionalized" to denote "age or time depth." Their mention of "institutionalized," and my inclusion of institutions as a key feature of deaf community/national sign language on the sociospatial list, show that these axes are not fully separable.

IMPLICIT AND EXPLICIT DISTINCTIONS

- Are users deaf, hearing, or both?
- What is the scale and type of place where people sign?
  - Is this place urban or rural?
- How many people in this space sign? What are their relationships, familial and otherwise? What is their relationship to people beyond this space?
- From whom and at what ages do people learn to sign?
- Are there deaf schools and formal institutions, and (how) are these the key sites of emergence, transmission, and/or use?
- (How) are homes and families the key sites of emergence, transmission, and/or use?
- How long have people been signing in this place? How has signing changed over time?

Sources: Goldin-Meadow and Mylander 1983; Kendon 1988; Branson et al. 1996, cited in Kusters 2010; Kegl, Senghas, and Coppola 1999; Woodward 2000, cited in Nonaka 2007; Nonaka 2007; Kisch 2008; Fox Tree 2009, 2011; Meir et al. 2010; Kusters 2010; Zeshan 2011; Nyst 2012, cited in Kisch 2012b; Nyst, Sylla, and Magassouba 2012 (also cited in Goico and Horton 2023); de Vos and Zeshan 2012; Haviland 2013; Green 2014c, 2017; Neveu 2019, cited in Goico and Horton 2023; Hofer 2020; Hou 2016, 2020; Goico 2020; Horton 2020b, cited in Goico and Horton 2023; Reed 2020, 2022; Kusters and Hou 2020; Hou and de Vos 2022; Goico and Horton 2023; Moriarty and Hou 2023.

Actions, Orientations, Consequences

The following table offers a summary of the kinds of actions and orientations that I observed among deaf natural signers' potential interlocutors. Most potential interlocutors in Maunabudhuk and Bodhe are hearing, so the table is organized from the perspective of a hearing person; other configurations can be extrapolated. The relational consequences column includes ongoing effects on the potential relationships among participants in a conversation or interaction using Goffman's (1981) framework, with modifications for the interplay of both signing and speaking: signer, speaker, and addressee. I use the term *overhearer* to include perceiving both speech and sign (as *overlook* and *overwatch* have the wrong connotations); and *animator* refers to someone who articulates someone else's words or signs.

TABLE A.4 Actions, orientations, and consequences

Action(s) taken by hearing person	Orientation(s) implied by action(s)	Material consequences	Relational consequences
+ Eye gaze in response to signing	Willing to engage, affirming of potential intelligibility	Sensory possibility of understanding	Meets the signer's bid for an addressee
– Eye gaze in response to signing	Unwilling to engage, denial of potential intelligibility	Sensory impossibility of understanding	Refuses signer's bid for an addressee
+ Eye glaze (eyes take on unfocused expression and sometimes move away from signer)	Unwilling to engage, denial of potential intelligibility	Various	Refuses signer's bid for an addressee
+ Signing (as first move)	"I can sign, the person I'm signing to can understand"	Initiates first turn in possible sequence of turns	Makes a bid for signer-addressee configuration with deaf person as addressee
+ Signing (in response to sign)	"I can sign, I have understood enough to respond, this person can understand me in turn"	Continues conversational turn-taking	Affirms signer-addressee configuration and reverses it
– Signing (in response to sign)	"I do not understand and/or this is not worth engaging"	Ends conversational turn-taking, constitutes a move by absence	Depends on other actions; often ends signer-addressee configuration
+ Speech indicating lack of understanding + Sign indicating understanding	"This is a person who I am likely to not understand even if I'm responding"; sets up possibility for disengagement	Speech and sign contradict	Affirms signer-addressee configuration and reverses it; makes bid for turn as speaker (other hearing people sought as addressees or overhearers); negative evaluation of ongoing interaction indexes negative evaluation of person's intelligibility more generally; reflects and reinforces a field in which neither engagement nor understanding are guaranteed

TABLE A.4 Continued

Action(s) taken by hearing person	Orientation(s) implied by action(s)	Material consequences	Relational consequences
+ Speech indicating lack of understanding + Eye gaze but no signing	"I do not understand"	Understanding is materially possible but evaluated as not occurring	Maintains signer-addressee configuration but does not reverse it; bid for turn as speaker (other hearing people sought as addressees or overhearers); evaluates signer as unintelligible in the moment if not more generally
+ Speech indicating lack of understanding − Eye gaze (or + eye glaze)	"I could not possibly understand"	Fulfills prediction of not understanding by making it impossible or difficult to do so	Refuses or ends signer-addressee configuration; bid for turn as speaker (other hearing people sought as addressees or overhearers)
+ Speech requesting translation	Affirms signer's potential intelligibility	Opens potential spoken conversational sequence (someone can respond with a translation)	Pauses signer-addressee relationship to make bid for spoken interaction, with potential goal of reestablishing signed interaction
+ Speech constituting translation (unprompted)	Affirms intelligibility while acknowledging others may not understand; may or may not naturalize expectation that some people cannot or need not try to understand sign	Offers spoken language rendition of sign (may or may not be "accurate")	Turns speaker into signer's animator
+ Speech constituting translation (prompted)	Affirms intelligibility; acknowledges that someone has requested a translation and that giving one is possible	Offers spoken language rendition of sign (may or may not be "accurate")	Turns speaker into signer's animator

Guide to Transcripts

CAPS REGULAR:	natural sign (or occasionally bivalent sign) glossed in English
CAPS BOLD:	NSL glossed in English
CAPS ITALICS:	natural sign glossed in Nepali
CAPS-CAPS:	single sign glossed by multiple written words
lowercase italics:	speech
Mixed-case bold:	English translation
[brackets]:	overlap in two or more adjoining turns
(parentheses):	descriptions of movements and actions
SLASH/mark:	links simultaneously articulated speech/sign
SLASH/MARK:	links two possible meanings of a single sign
plus sign+:	repetition of immediately preceding sign(s)
Point-word:	point followed by the person, place, object, or direction pointed at
Q:	natural sign that serves as general wh-question
NEG:	natural sign that has negating function
(?):	gloss of preceding sign is tentative
###:	signs that I do not know how to gloss
%%:	speech I cannot hear clearly enough to transcribe, even tentatively

For spoken and written Nepali, I use the International Alphabet of Sanskrit Transliteration (IAST), with the following modifications, most of which are common among Nepal scholars:

VOWELS

I do not differentiate between long and short *i* and *u*.
ā and *a* correspond to two distinct phonemes.
I write *x̃* for nasalized vowels, where *x* is any vowel.

CONSONANTS

I write *sh* for *ś* and *ṣ*.
I write *ch* for *c* and *chh* for *ch*.
I write *ng* for *ṅ* and *ṅg*.
I write *w* for *v*.

Transcripts

Numbered lines indicate turns; line breaks within turns are for ease of reading.

CHAPTER 4: VIDEO JUNE 18, 2010[1]

Time code: 10:05–10:18

1	Krishna:	(responding to Sagar off camera)
		Point-self? Point-neighbor?
		Me? Him?
2	Sagar:	(signs something off camera)
3	Krishna:	(affirmative head tilt) Point-neighbor?
		(questioning head thrust, touches neighbor's shoulder) Q? TALK-WITH?
		(laughs, touches neighbor's shoulder)
		Yeah. Him? What am I supposed to do? We should talk?
4	Neighbor:	(turns to look at Krishna)
5	Krishna:	TALK-WITH Point-Sagar Q (laughing, patting neighbor on shoulder)
		So he says we should talk.
6	Neighbor:	(looks away, perhaps toward Samman) SPEAK NEG (looks toward Krishna)
		I don't know how to speak (sign); or, I don't know what to say
7	Krishna:	(side-hugs neighbor)

Time code: 19:59–20:07

| 8 | Neighbor: | (looking at forge) |

9   Krishna: (presumably in response to Sagar) Point-neighbor+?
                 (turns to Neighbor, briefly rests hand on neighbor's thigh) Q? (laughs)
                 [TALK-WITH Point-neighbor Q Point-Sagar Q]
                 Him? Hunh? He says we're supposed to talk I guess, how about that!

10 Neighbor: [(turns to look at Krishna)]

Time code: 21:02–21:35

11 Krishna: (turns to neighbor) SACRED-THREAD [Q? THROW-AWAY Point-
                 neighbor (laughs, pats neighbor's thigh)]
                 Your sacred thread? You've thrown it away.

12 Neighbor: [(turns to look at Krishna)]

13 Mara: *bujhnubhayo?*
                 Do/did you understand?

14 Neighbor: (looking at Samman) *ma ta hātko ishārā ta bujhdina ta*
                 I don't understand hand signs.

15 Samman: *tyo bāni ho*
                 It's habit.

16 Neighbor: *eutā eutā āūdāina* [*ma ta mmm* (looks down)]
                 I don't get even one little thing, I'm like—nothing.

17 Krishna: ([looks at neighbor, pats neighbor's knee, laughs], [squeezes neighbor's knee])

18 Neighbor: ([looks at Krishna])

19 Krishna: (glances down, looks at neighbor)

20 Mara: (taps Krishna)
                 Hey.

21 Samman: (looks at Mara)

22 Krishna: (looks at Mara)

23 Mara: **AGAIN UNDERSTAND** NEG SACRED-THREAD THROW-AWAY/
                 SIGN-TO-neighbor
                 He didn't understand, tell him again.

24 Neighbor: (looks at Mara part way through prior turn, then looks at Krishna as
                 Krishna begins to sign)

25 Krishna: SACRED-THREAD [THROW-AWAY]
                 You threw away your sacred thread.

26 Nephew: ([looks at Krishna])

27 Neighbor: (looks at Samman) *ke bhaneko?*
                 What did he say?

28 Nephew: (looks down at task)

29 Samman: *khoi maile pani bujh* [*dina, janāiko kurā garchha*]
                 I don't understand either, he's talking about sacred threads.

30 Nephew: ([looks up at Krishna, questioning head nod])
                 What?

31 Krishna: SACRED-THREAD? THROW-AWAY
                 The sacred thread? You/he threw it away.

32 Neighbor: (looks at Krishna)
33 Samman: *eh janāi [phālera]*—
    Throwing away the sacred thread—
34 Nephew: *[janāi] phukālera*—(general laughter)
    (You) took off the sacred thread—
35 Samman: (points at neighbor) *tapāĩko janāi phukālera phāldine bhanchha tyo*
    (points at Krishna)
    He says you took your thread off and threw it away.

Time code: 21:58–22:14

36 Neighbor: (touches Krishna's arm) SACRED-THREAD/*mero*
    [NEG/*chhaina* (touches Krishna's arm)]
    I don't wear a sacred thread.
37 Krishna: [(responding to something Sagar's said) [**PIG?** PIG], **PIG** Point-Sagar
    Pig? You (eat) pig.
38 Samman: (to Krishna) HEY Point-neighbor
    He wants you.
39 Krishna: [(looks immediately at neighbor)]
40 Neighbor: [(touches Krishna)] SACRED-THREAD NEG
    Hey, I don't wear a sacred thread.
41 Krishna: (negative head shake)
    No?
42 Neighbor: NEG
    No.
43 Krishna: [THROW-AWAY]
    You threw it away.
44 Neighbor: [FINISH]
    Gone!
45 Krishna: (touches chest) THROW-AWAY
    You threw it away.
46 Both: (laughing)
47 Krishna: *JEṬHĀ* 'OLDEST' (sign directed downhill) SACRED-THREAD *JEṬHĀ*
    'OLDEST'(sign directed downhill)
    Your oldest brother wears one.
48 Neighbor: Point-self/*hāmro JEṬHĀ* 'OLDEST'/*jeṭho?*
    Our oldest brother?
49 Krishna: (affirmative head nod)
    Yes
50 Neighbor: SACRED-THREAD/*chha?*
    He wears it?
51 Krishna: (affirmative head tilt)
    Yes.
52 Neighbor: (laughs, looks at Samman, back at Krishna)

Time code: 23:15–24:02

53 Krishna: (looking away) Q (looking at Sagar, gives questioning head thrust)
            NEG (looking away in disgust) *LOPPĀ* 'TO-HELL-WITH-ME.'
            (general laughter) NEG
            There you go. What? No, gross. How insulting! No.
54 Mara: DOG SAY Point-Sagar? DOG SAY Point-Sagar?
            Did he say dog?
55 Krishna: (affirmative head nod). ANIMAL (classifier) DOG EAT NEG
            Yes. I do not eat dog.
56 Neighbor: (touches Krishna) DOG EAT Point-self (general laughter, rather raucous)
            Hey. I eat dog.
57 Krishna: (playfully shoves neighbor, laughter continues)
58 Krishna: FINISH NEG, [EAT NEG]
            No you don't! You don't eat dog.
59 Mara: [*ke bhanubhayo?*]
            What did you say?
60 Neighbor: *eh kukur pani khāīdinchhu bhaneko* (general laughter)
            Oh I said I absolutely eat dog.
61 Mara: (to Sagar) [Point-neighbor **EAT-UP+** Point-self Point-neighbor]
            He said, "I eat dog right up!"
62 Samman: [*yo* (pauses)] *Indiāko ko ki jātharule che* [*khānchha yo kukur pani*]
            So . . . in India one of the castes eats dog.
63 Neighbor: [(touches Krishna) DOG NEG Point-Krishna?]
            What, you don't eat dog?
64 Krishna: (look of disgust) NEG
            No.
65 Neighbor: Point-self Point-up/away EXIST (sign directed toward direction of point)
            DOG HOLD SLAUGHTER OVER-THERE
            When I was over there, they slaughter dogs there.
66 Krishna: ABROAD+?
            You mean abroad?
67 Neighbor: (affirmative nod) ABROAD, EAT
            Yes, they eat dog abroad.
68 Krishna: EAT NEG
            I/they don't eat dog.
69 Neighbor: HORNS/*goru*[2]
            And this animal (in speech: bull)
70 Krishna: HORNS?
            What kind of animal?
71 Neighbor: *gāilai ke bhanchha?*
            What do you call a cow?
72 Samman: HORNS *gāilai yaso*/MILK COW [MILK/*yaso*]
            You sign cow like this.

73   Neighbor: [*eh*/MILK] (touches Krishna) *yaso*/MILK EAT/*khānchhan*
SLAUGHTER CUT-ACROSS-THROAT
Oh like that. They eat cows too, they slaughter them by cutting their throats.

74   Krishna: Q?
Yeah?

75   Neighbor: CUT-BACK-OF-NECK NEG CUT-ACROSS-THROAT. ABROAD.
Yes, they won't cut them on the back of the neck, only on the throat.
That's what they do abroad.

CHAPTER 5: VIDEO JUNE 16, 2010

Time code: 1:52–2:29

1   Mara: HEY HOME Point-Parvati HOME++ Q?
Hey Parvati, where do you live?

2   Parvati: Point-self Point-downward
I live here!

3   Mara: Point-downward
Here

4   Parvati: (emphatic head nod)
Yes

5   Mara: OLD-PERSON+ Q?
And your husband?

6   Parvati: MAN++ PAST (?) OLD-PERSON Point-downward Point-self
MAN WALK-LIKE-THIS Point-downward
My husband—the man who walked with a limp—lived here.

7   Mara: WALK-LIKE-THIS+?
Walked like this—oh with a limp?

8   Parvati: (demonstrate pronounced limp with foot)
BIRTH *MĀILĀ* 'SECOND-OLDEST', BIRTH *JEṬHĀ* 'OLDEST'—
A limp like this. I gave birth to my middle son, to my oldest son—

9   Mara: [*JEṬHĀ* 'OLDEST' Q?]
Where's your oldest son?

10   Parvati: [*KĀNCHĀ* 'YOUNGEST']
JEṬHĀ 'OLDEST' Point-downhill (grazes side of own head with hand)
Point-Shrila (touches Shrila) *JEṬHĀ* 'OLDEST' Point-downhill
and to my youngest son. My oldest son (unclear). Shrila and my oldest (son), downhill—

11   Mara: [(grazes side of own head with hand) Q?]
What was this sign?

12   Parvati: [HIT-self] HIT-self³ Point-downhill
I was hit downhill/someone (from) downhill hit me

13   Mara: Point-downhill Q?
What about downhill?

14	Parvati:	HIT-self HIT-self **I was hit/someone hit me.**
15	Mara:	Q? **What?**
16	Parvati:	### HOUSE FALL-OPEN [FALL-OVER HIT LEAVE (?)] **The house fell apart, tumbled down. Someone hit someone and left (?).**

Time code: 2:41–3:28

17	Mara:	HEY-Parvati Point-downhill Q? **So what about downhill?**
18	Parvati:	### HAT [HIT-self HIT-self Point-downhill] **(unclear) A man hit me. Downhill.**
19	Mara:	[Point-Parvati?] **You?**
20	Shrila:	[HEY-Mara Point-downhill/*u yahã* HEY-Mara] **Mara, downhill, over here—Mara!**
21	Mara:	[Point-downhill] **Downhill there**
22	Parvati:	[GRAIN-ALCOHOL] DRINK GRAIN-ALCOHOL DRINK HIT-self HIT-self GRAB-Shrila SHOVE-downwards/to the side **Someone with a relationship to alcohol hit me.** **He grabbed me and shoved me/I grabbed him and shoved him.**
23	Mara:	[MALE?] **A man?**
24	Parvati:	[Point-self CRY] **I cried.**
25	Mara:	Point-Parvati MALE [Point-Parvati]? **Your man (husband)?**
26	Parvati:	(affirmative head nod) **Yes**
27	Mara:	MARRIAGE? **Your husband?**
28	Parvati:	(nodding) **Yeah**
29	Mara:	HIT-self HIT-self? **Hit your face?**
30	Parvati:	(nodding) **Yeah**
31	Mara:	Point-Parvati MAN MARRIAGE? **Your husband??**
32	Parvati:	Point-self MALE WALK-LIKE-THIS (releasing/throwing movement) MALE (touches the porch) HOUSE. MALE *JEṬHĀ* 'OLDEST' Point-downhill HOUSE HIT HIT

		My husband who walked with a limp (unclear). The oldest here at the house . . . There was hitting.
33	Mara:	Point-Parvati MALE *JEṬHĀ* 'OLDEST'? **The man you're talking about is the oldest?**
34	Parvati:	Point-self *JEṬHĀ* 'OLDEST' HIT-self NEG **My oldest (son or husband) didn't/doesn't hit me.**
35	Mara:	[*JEṬHĀ* 'OLDEST' HIT-self] NEG **He didn't/doesn't hit you.**
36	Parvati:	[*JEṬHĀ* 'OLDEST' HIT-self NEG] **He didn't/doesn't hit me.**
37	Mara:	Point-Parvati *MĀILĀ* 'SECOND' HIT-self? HIT-self? **Does your second-oldest son hit you?**
38	Parvati:	Point-downhill GRAIN-ALCOHOL HIT-self HIT-self [SHOVE] **The person from downhill, the alcohol drinker, hit and shoved me!**
39	Mara:	[GRAIN-ALCOHOL]? **What's this sign?**
40	Sagar:	(makes noise from off-screen to get Mara's attention) **Hey—**
41	Parvati:	GRAIN-ALCOHOL, GRAIN-ALCOHOL (other variant of sign) DRINK **Grain alcohol—you drink it.**

Time code: 5:10–5:35

42	Mara:	HEY-Parvati (begins to turn downhill) MALE GRAIN-ALCOHOL Q? **Hey Parvati, what about the alcohol drinking man (from downhill)?**
43	Parvati:	Point-downhill FOUR (points to two other locations) FOUR. CARRY-ON-BACK COME-this-way ### (indicates foundation and walls?) (points to a fourth location) EARTHQUAKE FALL-APART **Down there, and there, and there. Four (places?). Someone carried something on their back and came this way. The house there fell apart in the earthquake.**
44	Mara:	HIT-self Q? **And the hitting?**
45	Parvati:	### HOUSE Point-downhill HIT HIT **(Meaning unclear; clear elements: house, downhill, hitting).**
46	Mara:	[Point-Parvati HIT?] **Hit you?**
47	Parvati:	[(turns body downhill) (grazes top of head with hand) *JEṬHĀ* 'OLDEST'] Point-self (grazes top of head with hand) *JEṬHĀ* 'OLDEST' *KĀNCHHĀ* 'YOUNGEST' (uses pinky of previous sign to touch Shrila) Point-Shrila Point-self *KĀNCHĀ* 'YOUNGEST' (grazes top of head with hand) *JEṬHĀ* 'OLDEST' HIT LEAVE DAMN (directed downhill)! [DAMN (directed downhill)!]

(Meaning unclear; clear elements: oldest, youngest/Shrila, hit, leave, downhill.)
Damn him/it! Damn him/it!

Time code: 5:36–5:50

48 Mara: (looks at Yug, nods head upward in a question)
            (implied: Do you understand?)
49 Yug: (shakes head, laughs quietly) %%
            (implied: I don't know, followed by something unclear)
50 Shrila: [Point-downhill %% *yahã* %%]
            Downhill, over here (something unclear).
51 Yug: [(sharply nods head upward in question) *ke bhayo*/Q?]
            What happened?
52 Parvati: (hand grazes top of head) (points downhill or to a fifth location)
            Point-self THIS-HIGH ### (walls?) EARTHQUAKE ### (bubbling up
            and crumbling?) FALL-APART (points at fourth location)
            (unclear) my child . . . in the earthquake the house that was over there
            fell apart.
53 Yug: (purses lips) Q? *thāhā bhaena malāi*
            What? I don't know.

Time code: 5:50–6:56

54 Mara: HEY-Parvati MALE [Point-Parvati]?
            Hey, Parvati, the man/your man
55 Parvati: [Point-Yug] (touching Yug) PREGNANT Point-Yug
            I was pregnant with Yug.
56 Mara: [Point-Yug]?
            With Yug?
57 Mara: HEY-Parvati MALE [JEṬHĀ]
            Hey, and the oldest?
58 Parvati: [JEṬHĀ?]
            The oldest?
59 Mara: [MALE *JEṬHĀ*]
            The oldest.
60 Parvati: EARTHQUAKE PUT-ON-BACK
            In the earthquake I put the oldest on my back.
61 Mara: (nods head)
            Okay.
62 Sagar: (gets Mara's attention from off camera)
63 Mara: (looks at Sagar) **UNDERSTAND, UNDERSTAND**
            Point-Yug PREGNANT [Point-Yug]
            I understand. She was pregnant with him.
64 Yug: [*bhanuhunchha*] *bhuichālā āudākheri* [*khoi*]
            She says when the earthquake came, that—

65   Shrila: [(taps Parvati) %%]
              (unclear)

66   Yug: *bhuichālā thāhā chha, bhukampa*
              An earthquake (lexical variant)—you know, an earthquake (lexical variant 2)

67   Mara: *unh, unh*
              Yeah

68   Parvati: %% FLOUR-GRINDER
              (touches Yug with both hands) PICK-UP ### (thrusts hands upward)
              I was grinding flour/we were by the flour-grinder (?)
              and I picked up someone and we left (?)

69   Yug: *bhuichālā āudākheri dājulāi bokhera lāgeko kahā̃ lānubhaera bhanuhunchha*
              She says when the earthquake came,
              she picked up my oldest brother and carried him off (implied: to safety).

70   Mara: *ani bharkar uhā̃haru utā basne mānchhe [le piṭnubhayo ki ke bhanubhayo tapā̃i %% bitra basnu- basdā] kheri*
              And just before they said that the person who lives down there hit someone/ something—while you sat—were sitting inside.

71   Parvati: [(points to fourth location) Point-Yug (touches Yug) PICK-UP GO]
              It was over there, I picked up my child and left.

72   Mara: HEY-Parvati MALE
              Hey, the man

73   Yug: *hoina %%*
              No.

74   Mara: *hoina, bharkar tapā̃i bitra basdākheri* Point-house
              No, just now, you were inside.

75   Yug: *unh*
              Oh.

76   Mara: MALE HIT-self HIT-self Q?
              What about the man who hit your face?

77   Parvati: GRAIN-ALCOHOL Point-downhill ### (shove? go off?)
              [GRAIN-ALCOHOL DRINKS]
              The man downhill associated with alcohol.

78   Mara: [GRAIN-ALCOHOL?]
              What is this sign?

79   Sagar: (gets Mara's attention and signs something off camera)

80   Parvati: GRAIN-ALCOHOL
              Grain alcohol/Limbu.

81   Mara: (looking at Sagar) HUSH (laughs)
              Don't tell me!

82   Parvati: LIMBU, LIMBU
              Limbu, Limbu (presumably Sagar has just signed the NSL sign for Limbu)

83 Mara: (looks at Sagar in surprise at Parvati's uptake of NSL sign)
84 Parvati: **LIMBU**, GRAIN-ALCOHOL DRINK
           He's Limbu, he's Limbu.
85 Mara: HIT-self?
           And he hit/s you?
86 Parvati: HIT-self HIT-self SWOLLEN-LIKE-THIS
           (puffs out cheeks, holds hands out from cheeks)
           He hit me, my face was swollen like this.
87 Yug: *khoi thāhā bhaena*
           Hunh, I don't know.
88 Mara: *thāhā bhaena?* (nods head)
           You don't know? (Implied: Okay.)

NOTE ON REPRESENTATION OF NON-ENGLISH

1. John Lee Clark in his Protactile Theory Seminar (pers. comm.) argues that deaf and DeafBlind people "speak" when they sign or use Protactile language. I do not disagree. The distinction I make in this book is for practical purposes given the ethnographic and analytic importance of communicative materiality and modality.

2. Slobin (2008:122) argues that it is "misleading to read an article written in English about a sign language from another country—say Germany—and find capital-letter glosses in German, as if DGS [German Sign Language] were a form of German." I share his concern that glossing conventions can perpetuate the myth that signed languages are merely versions of spoken languages. At the same time, offering glosses in Nepali highlights important semantic, syntactic, pragmatic, and metalinguistic links across modalities and languages (e.g., Green 2009), albeit at the risk of erasing links between NSL and natural/local sign, on the one hand, and spoken languages other than Nepali, on the other.

Rosenthal (2009) analyzes the stakes involved in various means of representing signed languages in academic texts. Green (2014c:2–3, 92–93, 113–114) discusses the intricacies of glossing, no matter the glossing language used.

INTRODUCTION

1. Fieldnotes June 4, 2010.

Ethnographic vignettes and video-based transcripts are endnoted with the date of my fieldnotes or videos. The absence of a date indicates that I have had to rely on memory. When quoting fieldnotes, parentheticals are from the original; brackets indicate additions. For quoted utterances, I note whether I recorded it in translation or in a way that preserved the uttered form. My use of both past and present tenses in ethnographic passages and video descriptions affords stylistic flexibility and makes clear that my research and analysis are historically situated in the recent past—neither timeless (Fabian 1983) nor long ago.

Names of organizations and places are real; names of people are pseudonyms, with exceptions: I use real names when quoting deaf leaders' speeches at public political events, crediting artists, and citing people in personal communication.

Pseudonyms have been selected to preserve social indexes to gender and *jāt* 'caste/ethnicity,' with some minor adjustments to maintain confidentiality.

2. Words like *majority* and *many* reflect statistical vagaries regarding deaf people's population and language environments (Mitchell and Karchmer 2004; Hou 2016:5). Green (2014c:177) reports on statistics for Nepal.

3. I hope for my work to be read as an ethnography of the precarity of language for natural signers, not as a normative equation of humanity with language. Disability studies and other scholarship has made the critical point that people who do not "have" language are no less human, although they may be treated as if they were (e.g., Yergeau 2018; Rutherford 2021). I am also in conversation here with Rebecca Sanchez (pers. comm.), who defines linguistic precarity as "the precarity that differentially accrues to peoples' bodies based on how we do or don't use language, as well as the precarious existences of languages that are stigmatized and/or in danger of disappearing" and notes that the term builds on and responds to Judith Butler's work on precarity, which while highly generative also naturalizes people as always and necessarily language users.

4. The idea that people (almost) never fully understand each other, that understanding only has to be "good enough" for the conversation to proceed, is ubiquitous in linguistic anthropology but took me a long time to track bibliographically. My thanks to Xochitl Marsilli-Vargas (pers. comm.), who asked Jack Sidnell (pers. comm.), who directed me to Garfinkel (1967). I am also grateful to Derek Baron (pers. comm.), who traced one iteration of the concept to Locke (1690, Book 3, Chapter X, Section 22): "Some gross and confused conceptions men indeed ordinarily have, to which they apply the common words of their language; and such a loose use of their words serves them well enough in their ordinary discourses or affairs" (1824:36).

5. I am reminded here of Katharine Young's (pers. comm.) invocation of a hand molded by the cup for which it reaches. Taub's (2001) explication of "image selection" in ASL, a conventional signed language, is also relevant, although her approach uses the framework of cognitive linguistics whereas mine is practice-based. Indeed, what I call immanent signs are also present in conventional signed languages, including NSL. For example, the sign for Tihar in NSL is similar or identical to the sign for Tihar in natural sign. The higher degree of conventionality in lexicon and syntax means that interpretation is far more routinized in conventional languages, though Graif (2018) analyzes how the potential transparency of signs affects NSL signers' communicative and political practices. As the literature makes clear, the iconic and indexical affordances of signing do not mean that signed languages are any less linguistic than spoken ones. Meier (1987), Thompson (2011), and Perniss and Vigliocco (2014) write about consequences of iconicity in (signed) language; Perniss, Thompson, and Vigliocco (2010) explicitly discuss iconicity across modalities.

6. My use of the term *refusal* is in conversation with but also distinct from its use in scholarly work on recognition (Fanon 2008 [1952]; Taylor 1994; Povinelli 2002; Simpson 2014). Both refusal and recognition as concepts require close attention to context: who is recognizing or refusing what, as offered or requested by whom?

7. I thank Jack Sidnell (pers. comm.) for this phrasing.

8. Hanks, Ide, and Katagiri et al. (2009) refer to their framework as emancipatory pragmatics. While invoking emancipatory pragmatics, I recognize that people's everyday understandings of natural sign are not always emancipatory, as explored in this introduction and chapters 1, 4, and 5.

9. Depending on circumstances, deaf NSL signers may also use speech, mouthing, lip-reading, and/or writing with hearing people.

10. My fieldnotes (July 26, 2010) quote a hearing person who differentiated between what he called "standard" sign language and "local" sign language, using the English words in quotes. I have adapted the latter phrase to *local sign* in parallel with the NSL NATURAL-SIGN and in recognition that what is considered a "language" is highly contextual. I also recognize that naming/not naming something a language can have real-world impacts: in this case, not explicitly naming natural sign a language could be read as devaluing the communicative practices of the people about whom I write; however, naming it as such could be used to detract from deaf activists' ongoing work toward fully accessible, NSL-medium education for deaf people. In this book my goal is not to determine whether or not natural sign is *a* language, though it is certainly *language*, but instead to think about *how* natural sign functions both similarly to and differently from conventional language. De Meulder et al. (2019), Kusters et al. (2020b), Hou and de Vos (2022), and Goico and Horton (2023) offer discussions of related themes.

On the concept of the *local*, I draw on Massey (1994), Hanks (2004), and Das (2007) to define it in terms of a series of interrelated characteristics. First, the local implicates both spatial and temporal aspects of social practice that are significant for questions of communication. Second, the local is both embedded in and emergent from context and relationships. The second dimension leads to the third: the local is a scalar, or relational, phenomenon or unit. Finally, the local by definition always exceeds its categorization. Green (2014c) further elaborates.

11. Many questions remain for future research as to what natural sign looks like in other settings in Nepal. Arjun Shrestha (pers. comm.) points out that reports exist of robust local signing practices in Jumla and elsewhere in Nepal. How to think about such practices—whether they constitute natural sign, local sign, local sign languages; or are best described by another term entirely—is an open and exciting question.

12. Kunreuther (2014:13), drawing on Butler (1997:34), makes the important point that "people do not need to turn around in order to be constituted as a subject of social ideology" and that nonoral forms of discourse, especially writing, also have effects. Yet it seems that both Kunreuther and Butler assume that those present, even if not hailed by the cry, can hear and understand it. Building on Kunreuther's insistence that the materiality of voice matters in complicated, ideologically inflected ways (2014:13–14), my goal is to analyze how spoken voices matter differently to deaf and hearing subjects, and more broadly, how scenes like this one suture core theoretical tenets to particular kinds of people and not others. And building on Kunreuther's productive point that readers may fill in details—imagining, for example, the quality of the police's voice—I stress that readers have diverse sensory practices and imaginaries.

13. What would happen to the people in Althusser's scene if they were deaf? Given the moment in which I am writing, it is probably unsurprising—but no less horrific—that the police hailing them might harm or kill them. Lewis (2014, emphasis mine) documents

cases in the United States where police have "brutally assaulted" deaf people "for what has been described *by officers* as failure to respond to officers' *verbal* commands, aggressive *hand signaling* or resisting arrest." The Autistic Self Advocacy Network (2017) and Alexiou (2020) also discuss how disabled people who do not respond normatively to spoken language are subject to heightened police violence in the United States and elsewhere.

14. My use of the term *BAHIRĀ SAMĀJ* 'DEAF SOCIETY' reflects my commitment to thinking through the historical and cultural specificities of Nepal, and is part of what Friedner and Kusters (2020:35) call a broader "proliferation of analytics" beyond the originary "deaf studies concepts of DEAF-WORLD and DEAF CULTURE."

15. Kusters's film on interactions between deaf customers and hearing shopkeepers is of clear relevance (Kusters dir. 2015).

16. The phrase "anthropology otherwise" (Restrepo and Escobar 2005) seems analytically related but distinct. Meek and Morales Fontanilla (2022) offer a branching genealogy of the term "otherwise" from an intersectional feminist perspective.

17. Kockelman (2005:237) further argues that the intersubjectivity required for semantic interpretation is itself a semiotic process. In this sense, intersubjectivity is the foundation as well as the achievement of interaction (Duranti 2010; Edwards 2021).

18. I read Hanks's (2005b, 1996, 1990) theory of language as both phenomenologically emergent and grammatically patterned as consonant with Das's (2012) theory of ethics as both intentional and routine.

What do I mean by *grammar*? Conventional form-meaning mappings and rules of thumb by which certain sounds or movements and certain combinations of those mean something to someone. Drawing on Hanks (1996:33–34), grammar is what allows an English user to differentiate between "boy" and "dog" as well as among "The boy petted the dog," "The boy kissed the dog," and "The dog kissed the boy." Every conventional language differentiates differently; all conventional languages have areas where things can be ambiguous, at least when compared to another language; and all conventional languages have ways of clarifying ambiguity if and when needed.

I also want to emphasize that engaging with someone is not the same as being nice; antagonism can be intimate. People may be oriented toward signing and treat signers in general or one particular signer as intelligible and still have a fight, argue, or be cruel, in sign.

19. Moreover, *emergent language, emerging language, language emergence*, and *emergence* as a property of language in use are related but not identical concepts.

20. Kasnitz and Block (2012) similarly argue that communicating with persons with speech disabilities requires "effort" and "willingness." Willingness is also critical in interactions across accents (Nagai and Everhart 2022), dialects (Rickford and King 2016), and languages (Canagarajah 2013; Green 2014a). Relatedly, DeafBlind signers in the United States have had to challenge normative hierarchies of senses and what Clark (2017) calls "distantism" to make tactility a valued mode of participation in life, a mode in which DeafBlind people themselves are willing to engage (Edwards in press). Reno (2012), Hart (2014), and Rutherford (2021) also offer accounts of communication by and with neurodivergent and disabled people.

21. Resonating with my argument that conventional grammar does ethical work (Green 2022a), Annelies Kusters (pers. comm.) theorizes that more conventionalized IS requires less moral orientation.

22. Humphries et al. (2016) make a related point about deaf children who suffer abuse.

23. Maunabudhuk hosted Peace Corp Volunteers from 1984 through 1987, in the early 1990s, from 1997 through 1999, and from 2000 through 2002 (Jill Chaskes Foster, pers. comm.).

24. Fieldnotes October 2, 2009.

25. Fieldnotes May 11, 2010, and Fieldnotes June 18, 2010. While the two locales are different in important ways, Kisch (2008) describes a related integration of translation into everyday communicative practices in Al-Sayyid, a Bedouin village. More broadly, Hanks and Severi (2014) offer an account of translation in anthropology and linguistics, while Kelley (2014) includes an overview of theories of translation.

26. I am grateful to Bill Hanks (pers. comm) for encouraging me to do this.

27. Oralism as an educational practice was made official policy by the International Congress on the Education of the Deaf in 1880 in Milan (World Federation of the Deaf 2010), but its contemporary manifestations are by no means confined to the West. As discussed in chapter 1, Nepal's first permanent school for deaf children followed an oralist model for a number of years. More recently, Friedner (2022) charts how cochlear implant infrastructures in India privilege sound and speech over sight, sign, and gesture.

28. Henner and Robinson's "Crip Linguistics Manifesto" (2023:8, 14–15) in particular highlights the challenge in "threading the needle": that is, fighting against deficit perspectives and the stigmatization of deaf and other disabled people's communicative practices as "disordered" in such a way that their theories cannot be co-opted to support "ableist structures" that, among other things, deny deaf children access to sign.

De Meulder (2019) also argues for the importance of sign while cautioning that language deprivation paradigms as well as other discursive tropes can frame speech and sign as either-or and erase the multiple ways that deaf people communicate. She suggests that rather than refer to deaf people who learn sign language past childhood as "late" learners, "new" might be a better term. (Interestingly, NSL signers use the sign NEW to describe deaf young adults and adults learning NSL for the first time.) De Meulder et al. (2019:895) lay out a related risk in analyzing deaf peoples' translanguaging practices: the possibility of erasing the effects of inaccessibility and "sensorial asymmetries," as if "all multimodal communication" were "equally accessible, or emancipating." Goico and Horton (2023), citing De Meulder et al. (2019) among others, discuss similar tensions in scholarship on home sign.

29. My use of the word *fragile* indexes but also significantly diverges from Goldin-Meadow's (2003) conceptualization of fragile versus resilient properties of language.

1. DEAF THEORY

1. Fieldnotes August 2, 2010, briefly reference this event, which happened months earlier; my account here is also based on what I wrote from memory in Green 2014c. Interestingly, Sagar did not seem perturbed by the implicit message that one could and should prevent congenital deafness when possible, though to be fair I don't know how carefully he read the entire wall of writing. Taylor (1997), as a hearing child of two self-identified Deaf Americans, discusses her own ambivalence about efforts in Nepal to prevent deafness.

Hoffmann-Dilloway (2016) and Graif (2018) also address the meaning and stakes of the term *lāṭo*. My analysis of the term *bahirā* is indebted to Graif (pers. comm. and 2018).

2. Acharya (1997) notes that a "deaf cultural association was established in Rupandehi" six years earlier but argues that KAD should be considered "a trailblazer."

3. Fieldnotes summer 2006, reproduced in Green (2007). The phrase "school *boys*" is instructive, as the kind of freedom to spend time together celebrated here was, and to some degree still is, far more common among men and boys than women and girls—which is not, of course, to say that women and girls have not been instrumental in the emergence and reproduction of NSL and deaf society.

LeMaster (1997); Chapple, Bridwell, and Gray (2021); and Moges (2018) offer accounts of deaf people's diverse experiences of gender.

4. "Introduction," National Federation of the Deaf Nepal, https://deafnepal.org.np/en /introduction-of-ndfn/, accessed June 12, 2023.

5. In Green (2014c:21) I discuss how the transmission of NSL within deaf schools, which occurs despite a majority of hearing teachers whose competency in NSL varies widely, critically involves peers, older students, and deaf teachers and staff. The Naxal school now hosts an NSL-medium Bachelor in Deaf Education, enabling increasing numbers of deaf teachers to get formally certified (although there are reports of pay discrepancies compared with hearing teachers). Snoddon (2019) offers a more recent report on deaf education in Nepal.

6. Hoffmann-Dilloway (2016) and Graif (2018, especially 51–61) also discuss the importance of deaf space(s) in Kathmandu.

7. Similarly, Hoffmann-Dilloway (2016:79–80) discusses what, following Narayan (2002), she aptly calls signers' "emplacement" stories.

8. Translated from NSL interview, video August 15, 2012. Here, Prajwal ties NSL to formal educational materials like posters, and to peer-to-peer instruction, a point of contrast with natural sign, discussed later in the chapter.

9. Translated from NSL conversation, video April 2010 (date unrecorded). This conversation took place between two NSL signers without my presence but with the knowledge that one of them was filming it for me. Note also Prajwal's equation of deaf people with users of SIGN LANGUAGE—i.e., NSL.

10. Figure 3 is based on several framegrabs—that is, stills from video—from August 15, 2012. All of Nanyi Jiang's illustrations were produced in an iterative and collaborative process. I shared with her the video images (or in one case a photograph and in another case an online image of a shirt), and we would discuss what to highlight; she would draft a drawing and we would discuss further. Her own creative practices sometimes involved asking another person to reenact the often-blurry original images. Rendering video stills into line drawings offers the people pictured greater anonymity, in line with using pseudonyms, and offers readers much more defined images. Some videos I filmed, while other videos were filmed by my interlocutors or former partner.

During my time in Nepal, I did not see NSL signers fingerspell "N-S-L" in the International Sign alphabet, which NSL signers frequently do use. However, the fingerspelled abbreviation "N-S-L" is something I see and use in conversations in the United States with NSL signers who are also users of ASL. Some NSL signers' lexicon also includes a sign that refers to International Sign; the sign itself is the IS sign that can mean INTERNATIONAL or WFD (Green 2014a:462n11).

In addition, NSL includes a conventional sign, which I gloss POINTING-SIGN, that highlights how deaf Nepalis who do not know NSL rely heavily on pointing. In contrast to

NATURAL-SIGN, the term POINTING-SIGN can be somewhat derogatory; while NSL signers do not hesitate to say that they use NATURAL-SIGN, I have only once seen someone refer to themself as using POINTING-SIGN to communicate with non-NSL signers.

Due in part to standardization efforts (Hoffmann-Dilloway 2008), NSL is generally mutually intelligible across signers from different generations, areas, and language backgrounds, although there are lexical differences and syntactic differences (Khanal 2013, 2012), and people often understand their own social group most easily. The most significant tensions I have witnessed around differences in signing relate to how heavily it is influenced by spoken/written Nepali (discussed in Green 2014c, 2003; and Hoffmann-Dilloway 2016, 2008), objectified by NSL signers with the terms LONG SIGN (more influence) and SHORT SIGN (less influence). Short sign is also frequently characterized as DEAF, as when NSL signers say that a hearing person signs DEAF SAME 'like a deaf person.' What NSL signers judge to be an instance of long or short sign—not to mention (un)intelligible—depends on the context, including the signer and addressee(s), as well as on the linguistic features. Generally, though, many NSL signers struggle to understand long sign, especially when produced by people who are not also fluent users of short sign.

While I have previously categorized both long and short sign as NSL based on NSL signers' discourse, I take seriously Arjun Shrestha's argument (pers. comm.) that this classification might be inaccurate from the perspective of descriptive linguistics. Even more critically, he argues that this categorization could be used to undermine deaf activists' efforts toward ensuring that educational and interpreting services meet deaf signers' needs and respect deaf Nepalis' language practices. While I remain interested in shifting local categorizations, I could not agree more that it is imperative for teachers and interpreters to learn and use short sign, and I am grateful for the opportunity to discuss these matters with Arjun.

On the topic of local categories, Reed (2020) provides a detailed account of metalinguistic terms and concepts among signers in Port Moresby, Papua New Guinea, including what they call "CULTURE," which as she notes has many parallels with natural sign. Hofer (2020) notes similarities across what Tibetan signers call "spontaneous sign" or "spontaneous sign language," natural sign, and CULTURE.

In a very different context, that of Maya standardization and Maya-Spanish interpreting, Rhodes (2020) addresses questions of intelligibility, language contact, and language ideologies.

11. Translated from NSL interview, video October 4, 2010. This is a different, and far more benign (even positive), meaning of *natural* than that ascribed by Graif (2018) to hearing people's use of the Nepali *prakritik* 'natural' to refer to deaf signing.

12. Interestingly, Peter Graif (pers. comm.) observes that signers also use the sign NATURAL-SIGN to characterize the signing practices of younger generations of deaf NSL signers, which can differ dramatically from those of the older generations of NSL signers and go beyond the officially sanctioned signs in dictionaries (as do, for that matter, the practices of older signers). I observed this use of NATURAL-SIGN once in a situation where I would have expected to see the phrase SHORT SIGN used, as the type of signing in question was being contrasted with LONG SIGN. In that long sign is strongly associated with (hearing) teachers, whereas short sign is associated with deaf people themselves, to describe young deaf people's own intragroup communication as natural sign accords very much with the sense of signing that is not formally taught.

13. Translated from NSL interview, video August 15, 2012. Furba is adept in ASL and may have been mixed in ASL pointing strategies, knowing that I also sign ASL, an example of calibration (Moriarty and Kusters 2021).

14. Translated from interview, video October 4, 2010.

15. Hoffmann-Dilloway (2011a) mentions NSL-natural sign bivalence; Graif (2018) also notes that NSL signers produce signs that do not contradict NSL grammar when signing with non-NSL signers. The sign meaning BAHUN/CHHETRI in natural sign only refers to Bahuns in NSL, and the general wh-question in natural sign is narrower in NSL.

16. Translated from NSL interview, video August 15, 2012.

17. Translated from NSL interview, video October 4, 2010. I have simplified the exact interlay of our overlapping signing in lines 4–6.

18. Translated and paraphrased from NSL interview, video October 4, 2010.

19. To the best of my knowledge, none of Sagar's former students became participants in the deaf association, but as discussed in Green 2014c, participants in the 2010 NSL class found it a valuable experience, and I have met active members of deaf society who first learned NSL in an outreach class.

20. Description from NSL political speech, video October 8 or 9, 2009.

21. Translated from NSL conversation, video April 2010 (date unrecorded).

22. Translated from NSL and recorded in English in Fieldnotes November 7, 2009. The NSL sign I have translated here as 'intellectually disabled' is articulated at the temple and initialized in correspondence with the Nepali phrase *susta manasthiti*.

23. Venkat (2021) argues that very often cures are not the endings they are thought to be.

24. I am very grateful to Kristin Snoddon (pers. comm.) for pushing me toward deeper engagement with this topic, including by pointing me toward Southern-oriented disability studies and directing me to the United Nations' Convention on the Rights of People with Disabilities, which affirms the right of disabled people to "services designed to minimize and prevent further disabilities" (Article 25).

25. Attributing sole responsibility for an important event or shift is a common NSL rhetorical device that reflects and narrativizes how, in a tightly knit, numerically small society, the actions of one or a few individuals can have enormous impacts. The story also shows the role that visuality plays for sighted people in formulating assumptions about who people are—a theme echoed later in this chapter.

26. Fieldnotes October 9, 2009.

27. Translated from NSL interview, video March 23, 2010.

28. Fieldnotes May 3, 2010. Thank you to Himali Dixit for helping me to figure out the Nepali phrase, which I had transcribed incorrectly in my fieldnotes, and for refining my understanding of what it means.

29. Fieldnotes July 26, 2010, and Fieldnotes July 27, 2010; quoted speech recorded in Nepali.

30. Fieldnotes July 26, 2010; quoted speech translated from Nepali and recorded in English.

31. Translated from NSL political speech, video October 9, 2009. For more on the specific ways that the concept of *āwāj* 'voice' operates in Nepal, Kunreuther (2014), and, in relation to deaf activism, Graif (2018) offer ethnographic accounts.

32. Translated from NSL political speech, video October 9, 2009.

33. Translated from NSL speech, video October 27, 2010. In NSL the subject is frequently dropped, as it is here in the original. I often translate statements about deaf people made by deaf people using the first-person plural, but since Sagar has just pointed to the village's deaf residents, the third-person plural seems more appropriate. The NSL sign used by Sagar that I have translated as intellectually disabled is the one described in note 22.

34. Translated from NSL political speech, video October 9, 2009.

35. I have taken the liberty here to use the word *lāṭo* twice whereas the translated version to which I have access uses *lāṭo* in the first instance and *dumb* in the second.

36. Video October 27, 2010, quoted utterance originally in Nepali; transcribed by Abinash Pradhan and me; translated by me, with assistance from Shristi Ghimire. The word *lāṭālāṭi* pluralizes and nominalizes through repetition and gender marking (Hutt 1997).

Mother-tongue languages are a critical site of politics and a powerful trope in Nepal; Pradhan (2020), Turin (2014), and Weinberg (2018) discuss this in relation to spoken languages, while Hoffmann-Dilloway (2010), Green (2014b), and Graif (2018:120–121) do so in relation to NSL.

37. This latter possibility reminds me of an encounter in a tea shop in Maunabudhuk where the NSL class participants would eat following class. The shop was also frequented by the usual assortment of residents and people passing through. A visiting hearing woman expressed the sentiment that Sagar did not seem *lāṭo*, and, feeling responsible for expressing certain deaf social imperatives, I politely asked her not to use that word. She defended herself, saying that she wasn't actually saying something bad about him, and another woman—someone from Maunabudhuk whom we knew well—agreed. I said that the word itself was bad, adding that Sagar found it upsetting. To my surprise, the local woman replied, "Can Sagar hear?" Later Sagar and I talked over what had happened with a third hearing woman, who criticized the other hearing women. In the course of our discussion she contradicted the logic implicit in "Can Sagar hear?" (and potentially present in the hearing teacher's comments in the main text) with this analogy: "Just because you're not seen doesn't make it okay to steal" (Fieldnotes August 2, 2010).

38. Translated from NSL, recorded in English in Fieldnotes November 19, 2009. Similarly, Hoffmann-Dilloway (2016:85) writes about a deaf man who had started to learn NSL as an adult, whom another deaf man, an NSL signer, calls *lāṭo*. She describes the latter as being familiar with the former's life story and way of signing but also as literally signing over him.

39. Translated from NSL political speech, video October 8, 2009.

40. Translated from NSL political speech, video October 8, 2009. These literal and figurative meanings are not confined to the Nepali context. In a protest in Bosnia and Herzegovina "deaf and hard of hearing people" marched to the parliament building with "banners that read 'We Are Deaf, Do You Not Hear Us?'" (*Sarajevo Times* 2013). In conversation with her deaf interlocutors in the UK, Robinson (2022) makes the inverse move, writing about "deaf-centered listening" to move beyond aural conceptions of listening.

41. Translated from NSL speech, video October 27, 2010. The ellipses represent several pauses: I was interpreting at Sagar's request and needed a moment to catch up, and someone in the audience was instructed to sit down.

2. TAXONOMIC URGES

1. Fieldnotes May 18, 2010, lightly edited for clarity.

2. I am also in conversation with work that does not use these terms, including Kuschel (1973), Kendon (1980a, 1980b, 1980c), Shuman (1980), Washabaugh (1980a, 1980b), Jepson (1991a, 1991b), Fox Tree (2009, 2011), Kusters (2010), Kusters dir. (2015), Hou (2016, 2020), Kusters and Sahasrabudhe (2018), Moriarty (2019), Goico (2020), and Reed (2022).

3. I use *deaf demography* as a complement to the concepts of *deaf geography* (Gulliver and Fekete 2017) and *sign language geographies* (Padden 2011).

4. Translated from natural sign, recorded in Fieldnotes June 4, 2010.

5. Fieldnotes September 22, 2010; quoted utterance translated from natural sign and edited lightly for clarity.

6. Moriarty (2019) makes a related argument in the context of Cambodia.

7. Fieldnotes June 2, 2010, lightly edited for clarity; following description from video June 3, 2010.

8. Hoffman-Dilloway (2016:4–5) also discusses various ways to refer to deaf people in Nepali.

9. Fieldnotes May 3, 2010.

10. Fieldnotes June 18, 2010, and Fieldnotes May 3, 2010.

11. Fieldnotes July 26, 2010.

12. Fieldnotes July 26, 2010, Fieldnotes May 12, 2010, and Fieldnotes June 8, 2010.

13. Fieldnotes May 12, 2010.

14. Fieldnotes May 26, 2010.

15. Fieldnotes October 9, 2010, quoted phrase recorded in Nepali, and Fieldnotes June 18, 2010.

16. Fieldnotes May 31, 2010; quoted phrase recorded in Nepali.

17. Fieldnotes May 3, 2010, edited lightly for punctuation and clarity. This excerpt points to how I did not always fully understand spoken communication in the field as well as to how I assumed in such cases that the "problem" was mine; I also tried to do this when communicating in NSL with experienced deaf signers. I believe this assumption is appropriate given that I was, and am, a learner of Nepali and NSL but also take seriously Bharat Venkat's point (pers. comm.) that assigning oneself the capacity for failure (Halberstam 2011) and denying it to others holds its own ethical dilemmas.

18. Fieldnotes July 16, 2010.

19. Fieldnotes July 31, 2010; quoted utterance in English translated from Nepali, quoted utterance in Nepali recorded in Nepali. I am not sure if the old woman was saying, "May they not be born," or saying what she thought God should say. My thanks to Peter Graif for assistance with this translation.

20. Fieldnotes May 12, 2010; quoted utterance recorded in English, translated from Nepali.

21. In recent years scholars have sought to expand the category of *home sign* and/or introduced variations on the term—e.g. "communal home sign" (Zeshan 2011) and "family homesign" (Haviland 2013). The work of Nyst, Sylla, and Magassouba (2012) is particularly relevant here. They point out that much of the research on home sign has focused on middle-class, urban families in the United States whose deaf children went to schools where they were told not to sign. Based on research with deaf signers in rural areas in Mali,

where there appears to be some degree of cross-signer conventionality, they suggest the term "rural home sign." Nyst, Sylla, and Magassouba's account is highly generative in its close attention to how people communicate, hypothesizing of intergenerational transmission, call for more research as to the relationship between hearing people's gestures and deaf people's signing, and rejection of population/number as cause. Rural home sign and the authors' approach to it have important ethnographic and analytic resonances with natural sign and my approach to it, as well as some key differences: natural sign is not only rural; Nyst, Sylla, and Magassouba refer to "variation in fluency" while I highlight the situated nature of (un)intelligibility and the role of immanence; and Nyst, Sylla, and Magassouba differentiate between systems and languages, whereas I draw a heuristic distinction between emergent and conventional language.

Neveu (2020) and Goico and Horton (2023) also discuss home sign beyond the circumstances in which scholars originally used the term, the latter offering a productive analysis of the concept in different contexts.

22. Fieldnotes June 1, 2010, lightly edited for clarity.

23. De Vos and Nyst (2018) make the important point that features of sign languages that are due to age versus other factors should be disentangled.

24. Erich Fox Tree (pers. comm.) argues that "professional sign linguists often assume sign languages are young and may even reject seeing or seeking evidence to the contrary because of the theories they hold." In contrast, Fox Tree (2009:325) describes the "indigenous sign languages" in Mesoamerica as "not only widespread, autochthonous, and ancient, but also historically related."

Interestingly, the NSL category SIGN does not seem to include co-speech gesture among hearing people. In fact, I do not recall conversations with deaf NSL signers about co-speech gesture directed at hearing people as a category; natural sign encompasses purposefully bimodal communication directed at deaf people.

25. Kisch (2012b) and Kusters (2020) explore the impact of national or deaf community sign languages on shared sign languages. Regarding questions of transmission by both deaf and hearing people, Davis (2010:182) writes that Plains Indian Sign Language (PISL) "most likely developed from the emergent signed language of tribal members who were deaf or with deaf family members; and, over time, members of the larger hearing community acquired it as an alternative to spoken language," elaborating it as it "has been transmitted from one generation to the next."

26. I thank Carol Padden and Wendy Sandler (pers. comm.) for an email conversation in which I began to articulate my distinction between emergent and emerging. Meek (2011:50) also discusses emergent meaning and grammar within the context of language revitalization practices.

27. Green (2014c:177) summarizes the widely varying statistics regarding Nepal's total deaf population; Hou (2016:5) writes about population statistics regarding deaf people in Mexico.

28. Yet Fortier (2009:61) notes that "the concept of *prākriti* . . . [is] also fraught with a negative valence of the *ābikāsi*, an undeveloped state of being," as in the comparison in the main text between *local* and *developed* fruit; Pigg (1996, 1992) and Liechty (2003, 2001) offer analyses of development discourse in Nepal. NSL signers value and positively evaluate natural sign, while also acknowledging its limits; Graif (2018) analyzes the

negative meanings of natural that hearing people assign to natural sign. Local hearing people seem both proud and at times dismissive of signing practices in Maunabudhuk and Bodhe. In other words, while the English (translation of the) names given by deaf and hearing people to this mode of signing may feel unrelated, their meanings within Nepal are remarkably convergent.

3. SEMIOTICS

1. Fieldnotes September 22, 2010. The NSL sign translated here as 'habitually' is *PRAYOG* 'USE,' articulated multiple times.

2. My thanks to Emily Ng and Hannah Chazin (pers. comm.).

3. Even in Peirce's (1955) exponentially triadic framework, iconicity and indexicality are relations between two components of signs: sign vehicles and their objects. Immanence, drawing on Kendon's (1980b, following Mandel [1977]) classification of ways that signs represent, insists on a three-way relationship among form, base, and referent.

4. I am thinking here of how Hanks (2005a:198) uses the phrase "rules of thumb" to refer to the "instrumental heuristics" people engage when communicating.

5. However, as Taub (2001:2–3) argues, scholars have also understated the role of iconicity—widely misperceived as less linguistic—as a strategy to prove the legitimacy of signed languages. Kendon (2014) makes a similar argument, following Wilcox (2004).

6. The photographs in this section are from my personal archive, taken on a camera used by myself, the NSL teacher, and my then-partner.

7. I am expanding here on Kendon's (2004:106) argument that conventionality and iconicity (a concept to which immanence is related but not reducible) are not opposites.

8. These images are based on videos from 2010. Both signs are also used widely by hearing people in co-speech gesture as well as gesture sans speech. As explained in the previous chapter, however, I do not frame these as pre-extant gestures that deaf people then incorporate into signing. Hoffmann-Dilloway (2011b:379–380) also discusses the sign NEG, which is one of several negating signs and strategies.

9. Edwards (2018) makes a related argument and provides an analysis of the concept of affordances.

10. These images are based on a photograph and a video still from 2010.

11. Meier (1987), Thompson (2011), Sehyr and Emmorey (2019), and Caselli, Lieberman, and Pyers (2021) address the role of iconicity in learning and/or processing sign.

12. Fieldnotes July 25, 2010.

13. This confidence is based on my observations, metalinguistic comments by deaf NSL signers and hearing people who use natural sign, and the radically different feeling of communicating in natural sign compared with my other language learning experiences, as discussed in the introduction.

14. In this context the potential limits of knowability are relevant not only to ethnographic methods but also to more formal linguistic studies. For example, I collected data of natural signers responding to visual prompts. If the same signs are used across signers to describe the same visual stimuli, one might argue that those signs are conventional in the linguistic sense, but there is also the possibility of a kind of convention of sign-making: a

tendency or disposition to create signs in patterned ways that draw on widely shared non-linguistic conventions of movement, association, and typification.

15. Here I draw on Hanks's (2005b:69) reading of Pierre Bourdieu, in which he "distinguish[es] three lines of thought joined in the concept of habitus," including "the Aristotelian idea of the hexis, which Bourdieu treats as the individual disposition that joins desire (intention) with judgment (evaluation)." My use of the term disposition is, however, somewhat more general.

16. Quoted from Fieldnotes July 26, 2010. Unfortunately I did not specify if my use of quotation marks around the word "guess" indicated that the speaker had used the English term or if I was translating from Nepali.

17. In spoken Nepali, birth-order terms are marked for gender: e.g., *sāilā* 'third-oldest boy/man' versus *sāili* 'third-oldest girl/woman.' In natural sign they are gender-neutral but can be combined with signs indicating gender such as BOY/MAN or GIRL/WOMAN. For the sake of readability, I (reluctantly) use the masculine as default and when context indicates it, and the feminine when context indicates it.

18. Video May 31, 2010.

19. Fieldnotes July 21, 2010.

20. Fieldnotes May 31, 2010. In my fieldnotes I wrote "Limbu? Nepali?" about Jyoti's speech, but I don't know if I meant that I wasn't sure which she had used or that I couldn't remember.

21. Fieldnotes May 23, 2010.

22. Eve Sweetser (pers. comm.) first drew my attention to mirror neurons. John Lee Clark and Charles Goodwin both make clear that embodied knowledge is not only of one's own body but also of others'.

23. Moreover, what counts as misunderstanding is perspectival; in many cases what I might consider a miscommunication would get folded into ongoing conversations and resolved through continuation, rather than through explicit recognition and repair (which would have provided me with less speculative data). And sometimes miscommunications were "resolved" with an evaluation by one person that another was lying or unreliable (analyzed in chapter 5).

24. Fieldnotes June 1, 2010. I told Sagar what Samman had intended to ask in line with the relationship of mutual interpreting that we developed both through explicit conversations about communication and through daily practice.

25. Video June 4, 2010; I have simplified the overlapping of lines in the transcript.

26. Fieldnotes May 24, 2010, quoted utterances translated from Nepali and recorded in English.

4. ETHICS

1. Translated from Nepali, recorded in Fieldnotes May 19, 2010. Even in the shared signing community of Adamorobe, "most signed interactions . . . between deaf and hearing peoples" are "short" in duration (Kusters 2014:145).

2. As mentioned in the acknowledgments, it was also important for me to think about why, when my then-partner, a hearing woman from the United States, came to

Maunabudhuk, she communicated both with Sagar and with deaf natural signers in ways that some hearing residents could or did not.

3. I argue that this irreducibility of the role of ethics is as true of settings like deaf schools or shared sign communities, sites for the emergence of conventional signed languages, as it is for places like Maunabudhuk and Bodhe.

4. I put the word *sighted* in parentheses to signal that default assumptions about deaf sociality and deaf persons as sighted frequently go unstated *and* that deafblind people do participate in deaf spaces that are organized primarily around visual practices.

5. Sirvage (2015) further argues that a signer watches their addressee, who is watching the signer, in part to monitor the addressee for indications that something relevant might be occurring behind the signer's back (dorsally). The signer trusts that the addressee will alert them if necessary, and it is this trust that enables the signer to freely attend to what they are expressing rather than to monitoring the environment for other cues about what is happening dorsally.

6. For blind or deafblind people, or in cases where direct eye contact is taboo, the absence of eye gaze would not signal or enact lack of attention. Clark (2017, 2023), granda and Nuccio (2018), and Edwards (2022) offer accounts of DeafBlind people's shifting norms around co-presence, intersubjectivity, and Protactile language practices. I thank Michele Friedner (pers. comm.) for first pushing me to deuniversalize the link between eye gaze and attention/orientation.

7. Fieldnotes October 17, 2009. In retrospect, I wonder if I used the sign COMMUNI-CATION in phrasing my question to Prajwal. COMMUNICATION is closely associated with NSL, and official framing, and sometimes deaf NSL signers' own discourse, positions hearing teachers' use of sign as NSL (Hoffmann-Dilloway 2008, note 10 in chapter 1). Perhaps these factors initially prompted Prajwal to say that communication wasn't the problem, but as the unfolding conversation shows, when teachers use LONG SIGN, they do not facilitate the deep understanding that NSL signers want and deserve.

8. Fieldnotes July 15, 2010. Binita Pradhan's pseudonym accurately indexes her relatively dominant caste; she was not a member of the Dalit subcaste often associated with tailoring.

9. This illustration is based on an image of a *cholo* that I accessed in 2014 from http://sarishop.com/zencart/images/shop/images/patterns/chololine.jpg but is no longer available.

10. Scholars debate whether signs should be thought of as interpreted in the mind. Kockelman (2005), for example, argues for a reading of Peirce (1955) that is less mentalist than my own, which I trace to the divergence between Kockelman's interest in thinking about semiotics broadly, including nonhuman semiotics, and my interest in thinking about specifically human semiotics and in particular the ethnographic phenomenon I'm calling *refusal*.

11. Fieldnotes May 12, 2010, and Fieldnotes May 15, 2010. Anthropologists now routinely acknowledge that anthropological accounts are subjective, partial, and situated; this is true not only because of what is often called *positionality* but also because of deeply personal relationships and investments in unfolding, ethically charged worlds. Put more plainly, my analysis has been viscerally informed by my negative feelings about Binata, which were shaped by our interactions.

12. In contrast, Kisch (2008) and Kusters (2014) describe shared signing communities where possible translators are in general readily available. Other research on nonprofessional

translational practices—both within sign and across speech and sign—includes Friedner (2015) on helping others understand, Green (2015) on informal interpreting, Kusters, De Meulder, and Napier (2021) on translanguaging (including brokering and mixing), Napier (2021) on brokering, and Kolb and Loh (2022) on "friendterpreting."

13. Descriptions and quotations from video June 18, 2010. For purposes of visual clarity, the image in figure 18 is based on a framegrab from ten minutes later than the quoted utterance. During our visits to the homes of the NSL class participants, Bhola often took on partial responsible for getting good footage. Relatedly, Hou (2020:667) offers an account of a deaf woman's insistence that her deaf sister take signing on-camera more seriously.

14. Fieldnotes May 31, 2010, and Fieldnotes June 1, 2010. Contradictions around understanding were not limited to sign. In early May 2010, Sagar and I went to the home of a deaf teenager, where we had the opportunity to talk with his mother. The teenager communicated primarily in Nepali, but I, as a non-native speaker, could not make sense of everything he said. I assumed his mother would be able to. At one point I directly asked her what he had said, and she replied: "I don't understand, I don't understand everything he says." She then proceeded to translate (Fieldnotes May 2, 2010; quoted utterance translated from Nepali and recorded in English).

15. Fieldnotes June 1, 2010. I likely used the adverb *purāi* 'completely' to try to show that I was interested in how much Samman understood rather than in a binary of understanding/not-understanding, although it could have had the opposite effect. In Nepali, speakers might say they understand someone *purāi* 'completely' or *ali ali* 'a little' and in NSL, signers often differentiate between being able to communicate in a language FULLY or PARTLY/HALF.

16. Fieldnotes October 10, 2010. In fact, when I asked hearing people questions like "Do you understand signing?" or "Do you understand your neighbor?" outside of the context of particular interactions, they usually answered that they understood or that they sometimes understood or "guessed." Such evaluations affirm that signing, or the signer in question, is potentially intelligible, at least to some degree or with some effort. I should note that I did not systematically survey people, and may have asked people who were more likely to engage with signers.

17. Fieldnotes May 24, 2010.

5. UNDERSTANDING

1. Kusters (2014:145, emphasis in original) observes that Adamorobe Sign Language "is only used by hearing people when talking *directly* to or with a deaf person, not in mixed deaf-hearing group conversations," which she suggests is typical of shared signing communities (155). In this respect, then, Maunabudhuk and Bodhe are similar to shared signing communities.

2. Fieldnotes May 25, 2010. Thank you to Peter Graif (pers. comm.) for helping craft a translation that preserves the original's formal repetition. Gender here is contextually derived, not grammatically indicated.

3. Conversations with Terra Edwards (pers. comm.) helped me articulate this question. Edwards and Brentari (2020) offer a compelling analysis of language and interaction in relation to Protactile, a language used by DeafBlind people in the United States.

4. Fieldnotes May 5, 2010.

5. I am reminded of a time in 2010 when I stopped to say hello to Sarita Nepali, one of the NSL class participants, as she was working in a neighbor's fields. She greeted me with a *namaste* and then announced to the people around her that I was there to yell at her for not having come to class. Trying to mitigate my perceived authority, which I wanted to reroute to Sagar, the actual teacher, and also to show that I was sympathetic to the demands of a farming economy, I told her repeatedly that I was not there to scold her. It only occurred to me a few days later that Sarita might have been strategically displacing her desire to go to class onto me (Fieldnotes June 6, 2010).

While she cited me as a reason to attend class, hearing people concerned about the labor lost when their deaf family members attended class sometimes cited this worry but also their deaf relatives' own needs as a reason for them to not attend class. For example, Sanu Kumari Limbu's husband came to class one day to complain that going to class meant she was gone too long, wasn't able to do work, and arrived home too hungry (Fieldnotes June 7, 2010). Padma's proud mother reminded us that he had been to school and already knew how to write, so it was embarrassing for him to sit in class learning the alphabet (Fieldnotes May 12, 2010). Like Sarita, Sanu Kumari's husband and Padma's mother invoked someone else as the locus of agency, distancing the speaker from the demand that the deaf person stay home to work. Ahearn (2001) offers an in-depth analysis of how people enacted and talked about agency in a Nepali village in the 1990s.

6. Description, transcription, and translation from video June 16, 2010. This section's title invokes Favret-Saada (1990).

7. The sign Parvati uses here and the sign GRAIN-ALCOHOL analyzed in chapter 3 are distinct, although for both the base is making alcohol and both have multiple possible referential functions.

8. At the time I was baffled by the introduction of the earthquake as a topic, but reviewing my fieldnotes later, I realized that in class that morning we had been talking about the earthquake that struck Maunabudhuk in approximately 1980 (Fieldnotes June 16, 2010). One of the locations pointed to (line 43) was where the family's house had formerly stood; after it fell apart in an earthquake several decades earlier, they had rebuilt it in the current place, as I learned later in the conversation.

9. Both the not-understanding and the partial understanding options complicate the claim that closer relationships yield greater understanding in signing practices beyond national/deaf community sign languages. Nonaka (2009) proposes that hearing people's level of signing competency can be mapped onto what she calls social proximity. Padden (2011:24) goes further, writing that "how often signers interact with strangers impacts the form and structure of that language. . . . When signers are with relatives and members of the same village or community, the context for language is shared, and a common history develops over time. . . . In the case of strangers, communication needs to be more explicit, and shared knowledge cannot always be assumed."

Understanding, signing competency, and language structure are not identical analytics, but they are pointing to something similar. In Maunabudhuk and Bodhe some deaf persons' hearing family members did describe themselves as able to understand their deaf relatives completely, and in fact as more expert than others. For example, Krishna Gajmer's twin told me: "We've used our hands to talk since we were small. Everything I say, he understands, everything he says, I understand. And other people would ask me, 'What did he say?'" (translated from Nepali, recorded in Fieldnotes October 9, 2010). As per chapter 4, Krishna's older brother concurred that understanding arises through habit. Yet here, even though Yug is Parvati's son, he may not understand (or understand enough).

10. I remember when a close friend, a deaf NSL signer, explained to her hearing brother, who was not an NSL signer, that sometimes she simply wanted to be together, even if they couldn't have a robust conversation. In Kusters et al. (2020b) my coauthors and I argue that in certain international situations, deaf signers prioritize the process of signing together over full referential understanding. Perhaps it is no coincidence that in both of these scenarios, the deaf signers are members of deaf-centered signing communities where understanding and being understood is frequently easeful.

11. Jakobson's (1959) definition of meaning through translation is concordant with Peirce's (1955) notion of the interpretant—although for Peirce the interpretant could be the same sign as the original and need not be "reworded."

12. Fieldnotes September 18, 2010, and Fieldnotes September 19, 2010. As I discuss in this chapter, Sagar often doubted the veracity of some local signers' narratives. Here Krishna was also annoyed.

13. Fieldnotes October 22, 2010, quoted Nepali phrase recorded in Nepali.

14. Fieldnotes October 1, 2010, quoted speech translated from Nepali, Fieldnotes October 17, 2010, and Fieldnotes May 31, 2010.

15. CREA (2012) states that they do not have "comparative evidence" to establish whether multiply marginalized women experience higher levels of violence but suggests that it is very likely. Khanal (2009) also documents that disabled women report high levels of violence (though again, direct comparisons are unavailable). Humphries et al. (2016) show that deaf and disabled children are more vulnerable to abuse and that deaf children who have been denied access to sign are furthermore "less able to report" that abuse.

16. Fieldnotes July 27, 2010, and Fieldnotes June 4, 2010.

17. In this series of examples the misunderstanders were primarily Sagar and me. I recognize the risks of laying analytic weight on examples that involve Sagar (who was raised in the same district but was not from Maunabudhuk or Bodhe), and even more so me (a foreigner). Although we were not long-term co-residents with years of shared histories, we both had strong investments in trying to understand local signers. Misunderstanding, moreover, is a difficult thing to pin down, as discussed in chapter 3, so it is easier to analyze in cases where I had access to metalinguistic discussions such as between Sagar and me.

18. Fieldnotes May 31, 2010.

19. Fieldnotes October 1, 2010; Uma Didi's speech translated from Nepali and recorded as indirect speech. It may be the case that most hearing villagers would have understood Jyoti as Uma Didi did. But Uma Didi was known by other hearing people as being particularly good at understanding deaf people, which I (and others) attributed to the fact that she lived close to Shrila and Parvati, though Uma Didi herself later told me it was because she had grown up with deaf neighbors.

20. Fieldnotes June 2, 2010.

21. I know multiple people in Nepal who follow prohibitions on food, drink, and commensality in their homes but not outside. As a mostly nonpracticing Jew, who knows other, more observant Jews who have different rules for different spaces, this feels very familiar to me.

22. Fieldnotes June 4, 2010.

23. Fieldnotes September 27, 2010, directly quoted speech translated from local sign. Indirect speech reconstructed from memory, as fieldnotes are on this occasion rather terse.

24. Fieldnotes June 17, 2010, and Fieldnotes October 23, 2010.

25. Fieldnotes May 26, 2010.

26. Fieldnotes March 23, 201, and Fieldnotes April 30, 2010.

27. Fieldnotes July 31, 2012, direct quote recorded in Nepali; food details from memory.

AFTERWORD

1. Snoddon and Madaparthi (2022:13) describe how for hearing parents learning American Sign Language, resources like pointing and handshapes (which, to be sure, involve language-specific patterns) can enable communication about things for which one does not yet know the signs. Rather than creating tension between a "grammar-focused" curriculum (2022:4) and an "action-oriented approach" (2022:13), Madaparthi (the teacher) emphasized "an open heart and open mind" (2022:9), mitigating parents' concerns about getting everything right, even in the context of learning a conventional signed language. Similarly, Marie (2020) shows that in Vietnam deaf teachers want to work with hearing interpreting students who can "OPEN-THEIR-MIND."

APPENDIX 5. TRANSCRIPTS

1. Shristi Ghimire provided transcriptions of spoken Nepali. Signed transcriptions and final translations of speech and sign are mine. For lines 14–35, much of which is hard to hear, I had input from Himali Dixit, Bicram Rijal, Abinash Pradhan, and Mark Turin. In Green (2014c:211), I explore multiple possible interpretations.

2. The sign that the neighbor makes in line 69 and the sign for COW that Samman makes in line 72 are very similar. It is hard to say whether in line 70 Krishna was saying, "COW?" or asking, "What kind of animal?"

3. When I repeat the gloss HIT rather than write HIT+ within a single clause/sentence, it indicates that alternating hands were used.

Acharya, Kiran. 1997. "History of the Deaf in Nepal." Translated by Erika Hoffmann-Dilloway and Durbar Chemjong. Unpublished manuscript.

Ahearn, Laura. 2001. *Invitations to Love: Literacy, Love Letters, and Social Change in Nepal.* Ann Arbor: University of Michigan Press.

Alexiou, Gou. 2020. "No Justice, No Speech: Autism a Deadly Hazard When Dealing with Police." *Forbes.* June 14. www.forbes.com/sites/gusalexiou/2020/06/14/police-killing -and-criminal-exploitation-dual-threats-to-the-disabled/.

Althusser, Louis. 1971. *Lenin and Philosophy and Other Essays.* Translated by Ben Brewster. New York: Monthly Review Press.

Autistic Self Advocacy Network. 2017. "Autism and Safety Toolkit: Research Overview on Autism and Safety." *Autism Advocacy.* Accessed September 29, 2022. https://autisticad vocacy.org/wp-content/uploads/2017/11/Autism-and-Safety-Pt-1.pdf.

Bahan, Benjamin. 2010. "Sensory Orientation: Part Two." *Deaf Studies Digital Journal 2.* https://doi.org/10.3998/15499139.0002.109.

———. 2009. "Sensory Orientation: Part One." *Deaf Studies Digital Journal 1.*

———. 2008. "Upon the Formation of a Visual Variety of the Human Race." In *Open Your Eyes: Deaf Studies Talking*, edited by H-Dirksen L. Bauman, 83–99. Minneapolis: University of Minnesota Press.

Bauman, H-Dirksen L. 2008. "Introduction: Listening to Deaf Studies." In *Open Your Eyes: Deaf Studies Talking*, edited by H-Dirksen L. Bauman, 1–32. Minneapolis: University of Minnesota Press.

Baynton, Douglas C. 1996. *Forbidden Signs: American Culture and the Campaign Against Sign Language.* Chicago: University of Chicago Press.

Bechter, Frank. 2008. "The Deaf Convert Culture and Its Lessons for Deaf Theory." In *Open Your Eyes: Deaf Studies Talking*, edited by H-Dirksen L. Bauman, 60–79. Minneapolis: University of Minnesota Press.

Bernstein, Katie A. 2016. "'Misunderstanding' and (Mis)interpretation as Strategic Tools in Intercultural Interactions between Preschool Children." *Applied Linguistics Review* 7, no. 4: 471–493.

Booth, Katie. 2021. *The Invention of Miracles: Language, Power, and Alexander Graham Bell's Quest to End Deafness.* New York: Simon and Schuster.

Bourdieu, Pierre. 1972 [1977]. *Outline of a Theory of Practice.* Translated by Richard Nice. Cambridge, UK: Cambridge University Press.

Branson, Jan, Don Miller, I Gede Marsaja, and I Wayan Negara. 1996. "Everyone Here Speaks Sign Language, Too: A Deaf Village in Bali, Indonesia." In *Multicultural Aspects of Sociolinguistics in Deaf Communities,* edited by Ceil Lucas, 39–57. Washington, DC: Gallaudet University Press.

Braswell, Harold. 2012. "Disability: The 'Difference' That Global Capital Makes." *Deaf Studies Quarterly* 32 (2). Accessed August 17, 2023. https://dsq-sds.org/index.php/dsq/article/view/3183.

Briggs, Charles. 1996. "The Meaning of Nonsense, the Poetics of Embodiment, and the Production of Power in Warao Shamanistic Healing." In *The Performance of Healing,* edited by Carol Laderman and Marina Roseman, 185–232. New York: Routledge.

Butler, Judith. 1997. *Excitable Speech: A Politics of the Performative.* New York: Routledge.

Cameron, Deborah. 1998. "'Is There Any Ketchup, Vera?': Gender, Power and Pragmatics." *Discourse & Society* 9 (4): 437–455.

Cameron, Mary M. 1998. *On the Edge of the Auspicious: Gender and Caste in Nepal.* Urbana: University of Illinois Press.

Canagarajah, Suresh. 2013. *Translingual Practice: Global Englishes and Cosmopolitan Relations.* London: Routledge Press.

Caplan, Lionel. 2000 [1970]. *Land and Social Change in East Nepal: A Study of Hindu-Tribal Relations.* Lalitpur: Himal Books.

Caselli, Naomi, Amy Lieberman, and Jennie Pyers. 2021. "A Threat to ASL Recognition or a Window into Human Language Acquisition?" In *Discussing Bilingualism in Deaf Children: Essays in Honor of Robert Hoffmeister,* edited by Charlotte Enns, Jonathan Henner, and Lynn McQuarrie, 35–47. New York: Routledge.

Caselli, Naomi K., Wyatte C. Hall, and Jonathan Henner. 2020. "American Sign Language Interpreters in Public Schools: An Illusion of Inclusion that Perpetuates Language Deprivation." *Maternal and Child Health Journal* 24 (11): 1323–1329.

Chapple, Reshawna L., Binnae A. Bridwell, and Kishonna L. Gray. 2021. "Exploring Intersectional Identity in Black Deaf Women: The Complexity of the Lived Experience in College." *Affilia* 36 (4): 571–592.

Clare, Eli. 2017. *Brilliant Imperfection: Grappling with Cure.* Durham, NC: Duke University Press.

Clark, John Lee. 2023. *Touch the Future: A Manifesto in Essays.* W.{ths}W. Norton and Company.

———. 2017. "Distantism." *Wordgathering: A Journal of Disability Poetry and Literature.* Accessed February 11, 2021. https://wordgathering.syr.edu/past_issues/issue43/essays/clark.html.

Clark, John Lee, and Jelica B. Nuccio. 2020. "Protactile Linguistics: Discussing Recent Research Findings." *Journal of American Sign Languages and Literatures.* https://journalofasl.com/protactile-linguistics/.

Coppola, Marie, Elizabet Spaepen, and Susan Goldin-Meadow. 2013. "Communicating about Quantity without a Language Model: Number Devices in Homesign Grammar." *Cognitive Psychology* 67 (1): 1–25.

Cormier, Kearsy, Sandra Smith, and Zed Sevcikova Sehyr. 2015. "Rethinking Constructed Action." *Sign Language & Linguistics* 18 (2): 167–204.

Creating Resources for Action in Empowerment (CREA). 2012. "Count Me IN!: Research Report on Violence Against Disabled, Lesbian, and Sex-Working Women in Bangladesh, India, and Nepal." *Reproductive Health Matters* 20 (40): 198–206.

Cuxac, Christian, and Marie-Anne Sallandre. 2008. "Iconicity and Arbitrariness in French Sign Language: Highly Iconic Structures, Degenerated Iconicity and Diagrammatic Iconicity." In *Verbal and Signed Languages: Comparing Structure, Constructs and Methodologies*, edited by Elena Pizzuto, Paola Pietrandrea, and Raffaele Simone, 13–33. Berlin: de Gruyter.

Dahal, Dilli Ram. 2003. "Social Composition of the Population: Caste/Ethnicity and Religion in Nepal." *Population Monograph of Nepal*, no. 1: 87–135.

Das, Veena. 2012. "Ordinary Ethics." In *A Companion to Moral Anthropology*, edited by Didier Fassin, 133–149. Chichester: John Wiley and Sons.

———. 2007. *Life and Words: Violence and the Descent into the Ordinary*. Berkeley: University of California Press.

Dave, Naisargi N. 2012. *Queer Activism in India: A Story in the Anthropology of Ethics*. Durham, NC: Duke University Press.

Davis, Jeffrey E. 2010. *Hand Talk: Sign Language among American Indian Nations*. Cambridge, UK: Cambridge University Press.

De Jaegher, Hanne, and Ezequiel Di Paolo. 2007. "Participatory Sense-Making." *Phenomenology and the Cognitive Sciences* 6 (4): 485–507.

De Meulder, Maartje. 2019. "Sign Language Rights For All, and For Ever?" Keynote presentation, World Federation of the Deaf, Paris. Slides and video. Accessed August 19, 2023. https://maartjedemeulder.be/slides/.

De Meulder, Maartje, Annelies Kusters, Erin Moriarty, and Joseph J. Murray. 2019. "Describe, Don't Prescribe: The Practice and Politics of Translanguaging in the Context of Deaf Signers." *Journal of Multilingual and Multicultural Development* 40 (10): 892–906.

de Vos, Connie. 2012. "Kata Kolok: An Updated Sociolinguistic Profile." In *Sign Languages in Village Communities: Anthropological and Linguistic Insights*, edited by Ulrike Zeshan and Connie de Vos, 381–386. Berlin: Walter de Gruyter; Nijmegen: Ishara Press.

de Vos, Connie, and Victoria Nyst. 2018. "The Time Depth and Typology of Rural Sign Languages." *Sign Language Studies* 18 (4): 477–487.

de Vos, Connie, and Ulrike Zeshan. 2012. "Introduction: Demographic, Sociocultural, and Linguistic Variation Across Rural Signing Communities." In *Sign Languages in Village Communities: Anthropological and Linguistic Insights*, edited by Ulrike Zeshan and Connie de Vos, 2–23. Berlin: Walter de Gruyter; Nijmegen: Ishara Press.

Delgado, Cesar Ernesto Escobedo. 2012. "Chican Sign Language: A Sociolinguistic Sketch." In *Sign Languages in Village Communities: Anthropological and Linguistic Insights*, edited by Ulrike Zeshan and Connie de Vos, 377–380. Berlin: Walter de Gruyter; Nijmegen: Ishara Press.

Desjarlais, Robert. 1992. *Body and Emotion: The Aesthetics of Illness and Healing in the Nepal Himalayas*. Philadelphia: University of Pennsylvania Press.

Dikyuva, Hasan, Cesar Ernesto Escobedo Delgado, Sibaji Panda, and Ulrike Zeshan. 2012. "Working with Village Sign Language Communities: Deaf Fieldwork Researchers in Professional Dialogue." In *Sign Languages in Village Communities: Anthropological and Linguistic Insights*, edited by Ulrike Zeshan and Connie de Vos, 313–344. Berlin: Walter de Gruyter; Nijmegen: Ishara Press.

Dirks, Nicholas B. 2001. *Castes of Mind: Colonialism and the Making of Modern India*. Princeton, NJ: Princeton University Press.

Dudis, Paul G. 2011. "Some Observations in Form-Meaning Correspondences in Two Types of Verbs in ASL." In *Deaf around the World*, edited by Gaurav Mathur and Donna Jo Napoli, 83–95. Oxford: Oxford University Press.

———. 2004. "Body Partitioning and Real Space Blends." *Cognitive Linguistics* 15 (2): 223–238.

Duranti, Alessandro. 2010. "Husserl, Intersubjectivity, and Anthropology." *Anthropological Theory* 10 (1): 1–20.

Duranti, Alessandro, and Charles Goodwin. 1992. "Editors' Introduction to 'Assessments and the Construction of Context' by Charles Goodwin and Marjorie Harness Goodwin." In *Rethinking Context: Language as an Interactive Phenomenon*, edited by Alessandro Duranti and Charles Goodwin, 147–150. Cambridge, UK: Cambridge University Press.

Edwards, Terra. In press. *Going Tactile: Life at the Limits of Language*. Oxford: Oxford University Press.

———. 2022. "Giving Up on Politeness: The Desire for Tactile Knowledge and the Art of Finding Life Lovable." In *Rethinking Politeness with Henri Bergson*, edited by Alessandro Duranti, 97–108. Oxford: Oxford University Press.

———. 2021. "Intersubjectivity." In *The International Encyclopedia of Linguistic Anthropology*, edited by James M. Stanlaw, 1–8. London: John Wiley and Sons, Inc.

———. 2018. "Re-channeling Language: The Mutual Restructuring of Language and Infrastructure among DeafBlind people at Gallaudet University." *Journal of Linguistic Anthropology* 28 (3): 273–292.

———. 2015. "Bridging the Gap between DeafBlind Minds: Interactional and Social Foundations of Intention Attribution in the Seattle DeafBlind Community." *Frontiers in Psychology* 6, article 1497. https://doi.org/10.3389/fpsyg.2015.01497

———. 2014. "Language Emergence in the Seattle DeafBlind Community." PhD dissertation, University of California–Berkeley.

———. 2012. "Sensing the Rhythms of Everyday Life: Temporal Integration and Tactile Translation in the Seattle Deaf-Blind community." *Language in Society* 41 (1): 29–71.

Edwards, Terra, and Diane Brentari. 2020. "Feeling Phonology: The Conventionalization of Phonology in Protactile Communities in the United States." *Language* 96 (4): 819–840.

Enfield, N. J. 2006. "Social Consequences of Common Ground." In *Roots of Human Sociality: Culture, Cognition and Interaction*, edited by N. J. Enfield and Stephen C. Levinson, 399–430. Oxford: Berg Press.

Erevelles, Nirmala. 2011. *Disability and Difference in Global Contexts: Enabling a Transformative Body Politic*. New York: Palgrave Macmillan.

Fabian, Johannes. 1983. *Time and the Other: How Anthropology Makes Its Object*. New York: Columbia University Press.

Fanon, Frantz. 2008 [1952]. *Black Skin, White Masks*. Translated by Richard Philcox. New York: Grove Press.

Faubion, James D. 2011. *An Anthropology of Ethics*. New York: Cambridge University Press.

Favret-Saada, Jeanne. 1990. "About Participation." *Culture, Medicine, and Psychiatry*, no. 14: 189–199.

Fisher, William F. 2001. *Fluid Boundaries: Forming and Transforming Identity in Nepal*. New York: Columbia University Press.

Fortier, Jana. 2009. *Kings of the Forest: The Cultural Resilience of Himalayan Hunter-Gatherers*. Honolulu: University of Hawai'i Press.

Fox Tree, Erich. 2011. "A Language of Slaves: Indigenous Signing in Modern Guatemala." Paper presented at the American Anthropological Association Annual Meeting, Montreal.

———. 2009. "*Meemul Tziij*: An Indigenous Sign Language Complex of Mesoamerica." *Sign Language Studies* 9 (3): 324–366.

Fricker, Miranda. 2017. "Evolving Concepts of Epistemic Injustice." In *Routledge Handbook of Epistemic Injustice*, edited by Ian James Kidd, José Medina, and Gaile Pohlhaus Jr., 53–60. Oxon: Routledge.

Friedner, Michele. 2022. *Sensory Futures: Deafness and Cochlear Implant Infrastructures in India*. Minneapolis: University of Minnesota Press.

———. 2016. "Understanding and Not-Understanding: What Do Epistemologies and Ontologies Do in Deaf Worlds?" *Sign Language Studies* 16 (2): 184–203.

———. 2015. *Valuing Deaf Worlds in Urban India*. New Brunswick, NJ: Rutgers University Press.

———. 2014. "The Church of Deaf Sociality: Deaf Churchgoing Practices and 'Sign Bread and Butter' in Bangalore, India." *Anthropology and Education Quarterly* 45 (1): 39–53.

Friedner, Michele, and Stefan Helmreich. 2012. "Sound Studies Meets Deaf Studies." *The Senses and Society* 7 (1): 72–86.

Friedner, Michele, and Annelies Kusters. 2020. "Deaf Anthropology." *Annual Review of Anthropology*, no. 49: 31–47.

———. 2014. "On the Possibilities and Limits of 'DEAF DEAF SAME': Tourism and Empowerment Camps in Adamorobe (Ghana), Bangalore and Mumbai (India)." *Disability Studies Quarterly* 34 (3). https://doi.org/10.18061/dsq.v34i3.4246.

Garfinkel, Harvey. 1967. *Studies in Ethnomethodology*. Englewood Cliffs, NJ: Prentice Hall.

———. 1963. "A Conception of, and Experiments with, 'Trust' as a Condition of Stable Concerted Actions." In *Motivation and Social Interaction*, edited by O. J. Harvey, 187–238. New York: Ronald Press.

Ginsburg, Faye, and Rayna Rapp. 2017. "Cripping the New Normal: Making Disability Count." *Alter* 11 (3): 179–192.

Goffman, Erving. 1981. *Forms of Talk*. Philadelphia: University of Pennsylvania Press.

———. 1967. *Interaction Ritual: Essays in Face to Face Behavior*. Garden City, NJ: Doubleday.

———. 1964. "The Neglected Situation." In *The Ethnography of Communication*, edited by John J. Gumperz and Dell Hymes, 133–136. Special Publication of American Anthropologist 66(6): Part II.

Goico, Sara Alida. 2020. "A Linguistic Ethnography Approach to the Study of Deaf Youth and Local Signs in Iquitos, Peru." *Sign Language Studies* 20 (4): 619–643.

———. 2019. "The Social Lives of Deaf Youth in Iquitos, Peru." PhD dissertation. University of California–San Diego.

Goico, Sara A., and Laura Horton. 2023. "Homesign: Contested Issues." *Annual Review of Linguistics*, no. 9: 377–398.

Goldin-Meadow, Susan. 2003. *The Resilience of Language: What Gesture Creation in Deaf Children Can Tell Us about How All Children Learn Language.* New York: Psychology Press.

Goldin-Meadow, Susan, and Carolyn Mylander. 1983. "Gestural Communication in Deaf Children: Noneffect of Parental Input on Language Development." *Science* 221 (4608): 372–374.

Goldin-Meadow, Susan, Carolyn Mylander, Jill de Villiers, Elizabeth Bates, and Virginia Volterra. 1984. "Gestural Communication in Deaf Children: The Effects and Noneffects of Parental Input on Early Language Development." *Monographs of the Society for Research in Child Development* 49 (3/4): 1–151.

Goodwin, Charles. 2018. *Co-Operative Action.* Cambridge, UK: Cambridge University Press.

———. 2006. "Human Sociality as Mutual Orientation in a Rich Interactive Environment: Multimodal Utterances and Pointing in Aphasia." In *Roots of Human Sociality: Culture, Cognition and Interaction*, edited by N. J. Enfield and Stephen C. Levinson, 97–125. Oxford: Berg Press.

———. 1981. *Conversational Organization: Interaction Between Speakers and Hearers.* New York: Academic Press.

Government of Nepal. 2012. "National Population and Housing Census 2011 (Village Development Committee/Municipality): Dhankuta." Kathmandu: Central Bureau of Statistics.

Graif, Peter. 2018. *Being and Hearing: Making Intelligible Worlds in Deaf Kathmandu.* Chicago: HAU Books.

granda, aj, and Jelica Nuccio. 2018. "Protactile Principles." Tactile Communications. Accessed September 6, 2023. www.tactilecommunications.org/ProtactilePrinciples.

Green, E. Mara. 2022a. "The Eye and the Other: Language and Ethics in Deaf Nepal." *American Anthropologist* 124 (1): 21–38.

———. 2022b. "Thinking with Signs: Caste, Ethnicity, and the Dual Body in Contemporary Eastern Nepal." *South Asia: Journal of South Asian Studies* 45 (3): 440–455.

———. 2017. "Performing Gesture: The Pragmatic Functions of Pantomimic and Lexical Repertoires in a Natural Sign Narrative." *Gesture* 16 (2): 328–362.

———. 2015. "One Language, or Maybe Two: Direct Communication, Understanding, and Informal Interpreting in International Deaf Encounters." In *It's a Small World: International Deaf Spaces and Encounters*, edited by Michele Friedner and Annelies Kusters, 70–82. Washington, DC: Gallaudet University Press.

———. 2014a. "Building the Tower of Babel: International Sign, Linguistic Commensuration, and Moral Orientation." *Language in Society* 43 (4): 445–465.

———. 2014b. "Language is Not Learned at the Mother's Breast: NSL as Deaf Nepalis' 'Mother-Tongue.'" Paper presented at Himalayan Studies Conference, Yale University.

———. 2014c. "The Nature of Signs: Nepal's Deaf Society, Local Sign, and the Production of Communicative Sociality." PhD dissertation, University of California, Berkeley.

———. 2011. "Beyond the Boundaries of Language?: 'Home Sign' in Rural Nepal." Paper presented at American Anthropological Association, Montreal.

———. 2009. "Nepali Sign Language and Nepali: Social and Linguistic Dimensions of a Case of Inter-Modal Language Contact." In *Proceedings of the Thirty-Fifth Annual Meeting of the Berkeley Linguistics Society, February 14–16, 2009, Special Session on Non-Speech Modalities*, 12–23.

———. 2007. "Slippery Like a Fish: Community, Ownership, and Nepali Sign Language." Paper presented at the Center for Race and Gender, University of California, Berkeley.

———. 2003. "Hands That Speak: An Ethnography of Deafness in Nepal." Undergraduate thesis, Amherst College.

Gulliver, Mike. 2006. "Introduction to DEAF Space." Unpublished manuscript cited in *Deaf Space in Adamorobe: An Ethnographic Study of a Village in Ghana*, by Annelies Kusters. Washington, DC: Gallaudet University Press, 2015.

Gulliver, Mike, and Emily Fekete. 2017. "Themed Section: Deaf Geographies–An Emerging Field." *Journal of Cultural Geography* 34 (2): 121–130.

Guneratne, Arjun. 2002. *Many Tongues, One People: The Making of Tharu Identity in Nepal.* Ithaca, NY: Cornell University Press.

Halberstam, Jack. 2011. *The Queer Art of Failure.* Durham, NC: Duke University Press.

Hall, Wyatte C. 2017. "What You Don't Know Can Hurt You: The Risk of Language Deprivation by Impairing Sign Language Development in Deaf Children." *Maternal and Child Health Journal* 21 (5): 961–965.

Hall, Wyatte C., Leonard L. Levin, and Melissa L. Anderson. 2017. "Language Deprivation Syndrome: A Possible Neurodevelopmental Disorder with Sociocultural Origins." *Social Psychiatry and Psychiatric Epidemiology* 52 (6): 761–776.

Hanks, William F. 2012. "Speech, Touch, and Gaze in Maya Shamanic Divination." Paper presented at the American Anthropological Association annual meeting, San Francisco.

———. 2009. "Fieldwork on Deixis." *Journal of Pragmatics*, no. 41: 10–24.

———. 2005a. "Explorations in the Deictic Field." *Current Anthropology* 46 (2): 191–220.

———. 2005b. "Pierre Bourdieu and the Practices of Language." *Annual Review of Anthropology*, no. 34: 67–83.

———. 2004. "Locality and Interaction and Interaction Analysis." Unpublished manuscript, University of California–Berkeley.

———. 1996. *Language and Communicative Practices.* Boulder, CO: Westview Press.

———. 1993. "Notes on Semantics in Linguistic Practice." In *Bourdieu: Critical Perspectives*, edited by Craig Calhoun, Edward LiPuma, and Moishe Postone, 139–155. Chicago: University of Chicago Press.

———. 1990. *Referential Practice: Language and Lived Space among the Maya.* Chicago: University of Chicago Press.

Hanks, William, and Carlo Severi. 2014. "Translating Worlds: The Epistemological Space of Translation." *HAU: Journal of Ethnographic Theory* 4 (2): 1–16.

Hanks, William, Sachiko Ide, and Yasuhiro Katagiri. 2009. "Introduction: Towards an Emancipatory Pragmatics." *Journal of Pragmatics*, no. 41: 1–9.

Harkness, Nicholas. 2017. "Glossolalia and Cacophony in South Korea: Cultural Semiosis at the Limits of Language." *American Ethnologist* 44 (3): 476–489.

Hart, Brendan. 2014. "Autism Parents and Neurodiversity: Radical Translation, Joint Embodiment and the Prosthetic Environment." *BioSocieties* 9 (3): 284–303.

Haviland, John. 2016. "'But You Said "Four Sheep" . . . !': (Sign) Language, Ideology, and Self (Esteem) across Generations in a Mayan family." *Language and Communication*, no. 46: 62–94.

———. 2013. "Different Strokes: Gesture Phrases in Z, a First Generation Family Homesign." Paper presented at Fieldwork Forum, University of California, Berkeley.

Henner, Jon, and Octavian Robinson. 2023. "Unsettling Languages, Unruly Bodyminds: A Crip Linguistics Manifesto." *Journal of Critical Study of Communication and Disability* 1 (1): 7–37. https://doi.org/10.48516/jcscd_2023vol1i ss1.4

Heritage, John. 1984. *Garfinkel and Ethnomethodology.* Cambridge, UK: Polity Press.

Hiddinga, Anja, and Otto Crasborn. 2011. "Signed Languages and Globalization." *Language in Society*, no. 40: 483–505.

Hinnenkamp, Volker. 2003. "Misunderstandings: Interaction Structure and Strategic Resources." In *Misunderstanding in Social Life: Discourse Approaches to Problematic Talk*, edited by Juliane House, Gabriele Kasper, and Steven Ross, 57–81. New York: Routledge.

Hirschkind, Charles. 2006. *The Ethical Soundscape: Cassette Sermons and Islamic Counterpublics.* New York: Columbia University Press.

Hodge, Gabrielle, Lindsay N. Ferrara, and Benjamin D. Anible. 2019. "The Semiotic Diversity of Doing Reference in a Deaf Signed Language." *Journal of Pragmatics*, no. 143: 33–53.

Hofer, Theresia. 2020. ""Goat-Sheep-Mixed-Sign" in Lhasa–Deaf Tibetans' Language Ideologies and Unimodal Codeswitching in Tibetan and Chinese Sign Languages, Tibet Autonomous Region, China." In *Sign Language Ideologies in Practice*, edited by Annelies Kusters, Mara Green, Erin Moriarty, and Kristin Snoddon, 83–107. Boston: De Gruyter Mouton; Lancaster, UK: Ishara Press.

Hofër, András. 2004 [1979]. *The Caste Hierarchy and the State in Nepal: A Study of the Muluki Ain of 1854.* Lalitpur, Nepal: Himal Books.

Hoffmann-Dilloway, Erika. 2021. "Images and/as Language in Nepal's Older and Vulnerable Deaf Person's Project." *Semiotic Review*, no. 9. https://semioticreview.com/ojs/index.php/sr/article/view/69.

———. 2016. *Signing and Belonging in Nepal.* Washington, DC: Gallaudet University Press.

———. 2011a. Lending a Hand: Competence through Cooperation in Nepal's Deaf Associations. *Language in Society*, no. 40: 285–306.

———. 2011b. "Ordering Burgers, Reordering Relations: Gestural Interactions between Hearing and d/Deaf Nepalis." *Pragmatics* 21 (3): 373–391.

———. 2010. "Many Names for Mother: The Ethno-Linguistic Politics of Deafness in Nepal." *South Asia: Journal of South Asian Studies* 33 (3): 421–441.

———. 2008. "Metasemiotic Regimentation in the Standardization of Nepali Sign Language." *Journal of Linguistic Anthropology* 18 (2): 192–213.

Horton, Laura. 2020a. "Representational Strategies for Symbolic Communication in Shared Homesign Systems from Nebaj, Guatemala." In *Emerging Sign Languages of the Americas*, edited by Olivier LeGuen, Josefina Safar, and Marie Coppola, 97–154. Boston: De Gruyter Mouton

———. 2020b. "Seeing Signs: Linguistic Ethnography in the Study of Homesign Systems in Guatemala." *Sign Language Studies* 20 (4): 644–663.

Hou, Lynn, and Connie de Vos. 2022. "Classifications and Typologies: Labeling Sign Languages and Signing Communities." *Journal of Sociolinguistics* 26 (1): 118–125.

Hou, Lynn Y-S. 2020. "Who Signs? Language Ideologies about Deaf and Hearing Child Signers in One Family in Mexico." *Sign Language Studies* 20 (4): 664–690.

———. 2016. "'Making Hands': Family Sign Languages in the San Juan Quiahije Community." PhD dissertation. University of Texas, Austin.

———. 2013. "Review of Sign Languages in Village Communities, Ulrike Zeshan and Connie de Vos (eds)." *Sign Language and Linguistics* 16 (2): 259–268.

Humphries, Tom, Poorna Kushalnagar, Gaurav Mathur, Donna Jo Napoli, Carol Padden, Christian Rathmann, and Scott Smith. 2016. "Avoiding Linguistic Neglect of Deaf Children." *Social Service Review* 90 (4) 4: 589–619.

Humphries, Tom, Raja Kushalnagar, Gaurav Mathur, Donna Jo Napoli, Carol Padden, Christian Rathmann, and Scott Smith. 2013. "The Right to Language." *The Journal of Law, Medicine, and Ethics* 41 (4): 872–884.

Hundley, Bethany. 2011. "Chasing Saraswati: Development of Deaf Education in Nepal." Unpublished PowerPoint presentation with notes, Fulbright Commission, Nepal.

Hutt, Michael. 1997. *Modern Literary Nepali: An Introductory Reader*. New Delhi: Oxford University Press.

Jakobson, Roman. 1960. "Closing Statement: Linguistics and Poetics". In *Style in Language*, edited by Thomas A. Sebeok, 350–373. Cambridge, MA: MIT Press.

———. 1959. "On Linguistic Aspects of Translation." In *On Translation*, 232–239. Cambridge, MA: Harvard University Press.

Jepson, Jill. 1991a. "Two Sign Languages in a Single Village in India." *Sign Language Studies*, no. 70: 47–59.

———. 1991b. "Urban and Rural Sign Language in India." *Language in Society*, no. 20: 37–57.

Jokinen, Markku. 2000. "The Linguistic Human Rights of Sign Language Users." In *Rights to Language: Equity, Power, and Education*, edited by Robert Phillipson, 203–213. Mahwah, NJ: Lawrence Erlbaum Associates.

Joshi, Raghav Bir. 1991. "Nepal: A Paradise for the Deaf?" *Sign Language Studies*, no. 71: 161–168.

Kasnitz, Devva, and Pamela Block. 2012. "Participation, Time, Effort, and Speech Disability Justice." In *Politics of Occupation-Centered Practice: Reflections on Occupational Engagement across Cultures*, edited by Nick Pollard and Dikaios Sakellarious, 197–216. Chichester, UK: Wiley-Blackwell.

Keane, Webb. 2016. *Ethical Life: Its Natural and Social Histories*. Princeton, NJ: Princeton University Press.

Keating, Elizabeth, and R. Neill Hadder. 2010. "Sensory Impairment." *Annual Review of Anthropology*, no. 39: 115–129.

Kegl, Judy, Ann Senghas, and Marie Coppola. 1999. "Creation through Contact: Sign Language Emergence and Sign Language Change in Nicaragua." In *Language Creation and Language Change: Creolization, Diachrony, and Development*, edited by Michel DeGraff, 179–237. Cambridge, MA: MIT Press.

Kelley, Elizabeth. 2014. "Translating the Arab World: Contingent Commensuration, Publishing, and the Shaping of a Global Commodity." PhD dissertation. University of California–Berkeley.

Kendon Adam. 2014. "Semiotic Diversity in Utterance Production and the Concept of 'Language." *Philosophical Transactions of the Royal Society B* 369: 20130293.

———. 1988. *Sign Languages of Aboriginal Australia: Cultural, Semiotic and Communicative Perspectives*. Cambridge, UK: Cambridge University Press, 1988.

———. 1980a. "A Description of a Deaf-Mute Sign Language from the Enga Province of Papua New Guinea with Some Comparative Discussion. Part I: The Formational Properties of Enga Signs." *Semiotica* 31 (1/2): 1–34.

————. 1980b. "A Description of a Deaf-Mute Sign Language from the Enga Province of Papua New Guinea with Some Comparative Discussion. Part II: The Semiotic Functioning of Enga Signs." *Semiotica* 32 (1/2): 81–117.

————. 1980c. "A Description of a Deaf-Mute Sign Language from the Enga Province of Papua New Guinea with Some Comparative Discussion. Part III: Aspects of Utterance Construction." *Semiotica* 32 (3/4): 245–313.

Khanal, Neeti Aryal (on behalf of Nepal Disabled women's Association). 2009. "A Study on Status of Social Inclusion, Livelihood and Violence Against Disabled Women of Nepal." Submitted to Action Aid Nepal, Lazimpat, Kathmandu, Nepal. Accessed October 20, 2022. https://scholar.google.com/citations?view_op=view_citation&hl=en&user=IJ6Q Mi4AAAAJ&citation_for_view=IJ6QMi4AAAAJ:UeHWp8X0CEIC.

Khanal, Upendra. 2013. "Sociolinguistics of Nepali Sign Language with Particular Reference to Regional Variation." Unpublished paper, Indira Gandhi National Open University.

————. 2012. "Age-Related Sociolinguistic Variation in Sign Languages, with Particular Reference to Nepali Sign Language." Unpublished paper, Indira Gandhi National Open University.

Kidd, Ian James, José Medina, and Gaile Pohlhaus Jr. 2017. "Introduction to the Routledge Handbook of Epistemic Injustice." In *Routledge Handbook of Epistemic Injustice*, edited by Ian James Kidd, José Medina, and Gaile Pohlhaus Jr., 1–9. Oxon: Routledge.

Kisch, Shifra. 2012a. "Al-Sayyid: A Sociolinguistic Sketch." In *Sign Languages in Village Communities: Anthropological and Linguistic Insights*, edited by Ulrike Zeshan and Connie de Vos, 365–372. Berlin: Walter de Gruyter and Nijmegen: Ishara Press.

————. 2012b. "Demarcating Generations of Signers in the Dynamic Sociolinguistic Landscape of a Shared Sign-Language: The Case of the Al-Sayyid Bedouin." In *Sign Languages in Village Communities: Anthropological and Linguistic Insights*, edited by Ulrike Zeshan and Connie de Vos, 87–125. Berlin: Walter de Gruyter; Nijmegen: Ishara Press.

————. 2008. "'Deaf Discourse': The Social Construction of Deafness in a Bedouin Community." *Medical Anthropology: Cross Cultural Studies in Health and Illness* 27 (3): 283–313.

Klima, Edward, and Ursula Bellugi. 1979. *The Signs of Language*. Cambridge, MA: Harvard University Press.

Kockelman, Paul. 2005. "The Semiotic Stance." *Semiotica*, no. 157: 233–304.

Kolb, Rachel. 2017. "Sensations of Sound." *New York Times*. Accessed September 4, 2023. www.nytimes.com/interactive/2017/multimedia/sensations-of-sound-vr-rachel-kolb .html.

————. 2013. "How Can I Help You?: Perspectives from a Patient with a Hearing Loss." *International Journal of Medical Students* 1 (2): 94–96.

Kolb, Rachel, and Timothy Loh. 2022. "How Deaf and Hearing Friends Co-Navigate the World." *Sapiens*. Accessed September 19, 2022. www.sapiens.org/language/friendter preting/.

Kraus, Kaj. 2018. "Deaf New Signers at Gallaudet: A Practice Framework for Deaf Conversions." MA thesis, Gallaudet University.

Kunreuther, Laura. 2014. *Voicing Subjects: Public Intimacy and Mediation in Kathmandu*. Berkeley: University of California Press.

Kuschel, Rolf. 1973. "The Silent Inventor: The Creation of a Sign Language by the Only Deaf-Mute on a Polynesian Island." *Sign Language Studies*, no. 3: 1–27.

Kushalnagar, Poorna, Claire Ryan, Raylene Paludneviciene, Arielle Spellun, and Sanjay Gulati. 2020. "Adverse Childhood Communication Experiences Associated with an Increased Risk of Chronic Diseases in Adults who are Deaf." *American Journal of Preventive Medicine* 59 (4): 548–554.

Kusters, Annelies. 2020. "One Village, Two Sign Languages: Qualia, Intergenerational Relationships and the Language Ideological Assemblage in Adamorobe, Ghana." *Journal of Linguistic Anthropology* 30 (1): 48–67.

———. 2017. "Gesture-based Customer Interactions: Deaf and Hearing Mumbaikars' Multimodal and Metrolingual Practices." *International Journal of Multilingualism* 14 (3): 283–302.

———. 2015. *Deaf Space in Adamorobe: An Ethnographic Study of a Village in Ghana.* Washington, DC: Gallaudet University Press.

———. 2014. "Language Ideologies in the Shared Signing Community of Adamorobe." *Language in Society*, no. 43: 139–158.

———. 2012a. "Adamorobe: A Demographic, Sociolinguistic and Sociocultural Profile." In *Sign Languages in Village Communities: Anthropological and Linguistic Insights*, edited by Ulrike Zeshan and Connie de Vos, 347–352. Berlin: Walter de Gruyter; Nijmegen: Ishara Press.

———. 2012b. "Being a Deaf White Anthropologist in Adamorobe: Some Ethical and Methodological Issues." In *Sign Languages in Village Communities: Anthropological and Linguistic Insights*, edited by Ulrike Zeshan and Connie de Vos, 27–52. Berlin: Walter de Gruyter; Nijmegen: Ishara Press.

———. 2010. "Deaf Utopias? Reviewing the Sociocultural Literature on the World's 'Martha's Vineyard Situations.'" *Journal of Deaf Studies and Deaf Education* 15 (1): 3–16.

———, ed. 2019. "Special Issue: Deaf and Hearing Signers' Multimodal and Translingual Practices." *Applied Linguistics Review* 10 (1).

———, dir. 2015. *Ishaare: Gestures and Signs in Mumbai.* Produced by MPI MMG.

Kusters, Annelies, and Lina Hou. 2020. "Linguistic Ethnography and Sign Language Studies." *Sign Language Studies* 20 (4): 561–571.

Kusters, Annelies, and Ceil Lucas. 2022. "Emergence and Evolutions: Introducing Sign Language Sociolinguistics." *Journal of Sociolinguistics* 26 (1): 84–98.

Kusters, Annelies, and Sujit Sahasrabudhe. 2018. "Language Ideologies on the Difference between Gesture and Sign." *Language and Communication*, no. 60: 44–63.

Kusters, Annelies, Maartje De Meulder, and Jemina Napier. 2021. "Family Language Policy on Holiday: Four Multilingual Signing and Speaking Families Travelling Together." *Journal of Multilingual and Multicultural Development.* https://doi.org/10.1080/014346 32.2021.1890752.

Kusters, Annelies, Maartje De Meulder, and Dai O'Brien, eds. 2017. *Innovations in Deaf Studies: The Role of Deaf Scholars.* Oxford, UK: Oxford University Press.

Kusters, Annelies, Mara Green, Erin Moriarty, and Kristin Snoddon, eds. 2020. "Sign Language Ideologies: Practices and Politics." In *Sign Language Ideologies in Practice*, edited by Annelies Kusters, Mara Green, Erin Moriarty, and Kristin Snoddon, 3–22. Berlin: De Gruyter Mouton; Lancaster, UK: Ishara Press.

Labov, William. 1972. *Language in the Inner City.* Philadelphia: University of Pennsylvania Press.

Ladd, Paddy. 2003. *Understanding Deaf Culture: In Search of Deafhood*. Clevedon, UK: Multilingual Matters.

Lambek, Michael. 2010. "Introduction." In *Ordinary Ethics: Anthropology, Language, and Action*, edited by Michael Lambek, 1–36. New York: Fordham University Press.

———, ed. 2010. *Ordinary Ethics: Anthropology, Language, and Action*. New York: Fordham University Press.

LeMaster, Barbara. 1997. "Sex Differences in Irish Sign Language." *Trends in Linguistics Studies and Monographs*, no. 108: 67–86.

Leve, Lauren. 1999. *Contested Nation/Buddhist Innovation: Politics, Piety, and Personhood in Theravada Buddhism in Nepal*. Princeton, NJ: Princeton University.

Levinson, Stephen C. 2006. "On the Human 'Interaction Engine.'" In *Roots of Human Sociality: Culture, Cognition and Interaction*, edited by N. J. Enfield and Stephen C. Levinson, 39–69. Oxford: Berg Press.

Lewis, Talila A. 2014. "Police Brutality and Deaf People." ACLU. Accessed September 29, 2002. www.aclu.org/news/national-security/police-brutality-and-deaf-people.

Liddell, Scott. 2003. *Grammar, Gesture, and Meaning in American Sign Language*. New York: Cambridge University Press.

Liechty, Mark. 2003. *Suitably Modern: Making Middle-Class Culture in a New Consumer Society*. Princeton, NJ: Princeton University Press.

———. 2001. "Women and Pornography in Kathmandu: Negotiating the 'Modern Woman' in a New Consumer Society." In *Images of the "Modern Woman" in Asia: Global Media, Local Meanings*, edited by Shoma Munshi, 34–54. New York: RoutledgeCurzon.

Locke, John. 1690 [1824]. *An Essay Concerning Human Understanding*. London: Printed for C. and J. Rivington, etc.

Lucas, Ceil, Robert Bayley, Carolyn McCaskill, and Joseph Hill. 2015. "The Intersection of African American English and Black American Sign Language." *International Journal of Bilingualism* 19 (2): 156–168.

Mahmood, Saba. 2001. "Feminist Theory, Embodiment, and the Docile Agent: Some Reflections on the Egyptian Islamic Revival." *Cultural Anthropology* 16 (2): 202–236.

Mandel, Mark. 1977. "Iconic Devices in American Sign Language." In *On the Other Hand: New Perspectives in American Sign Language*, edited by Lynn A. Friedman, 57–107. London: Academic Press.

Marie, Aron S. 2020. "Finding Interpreters Who Can 'OPEN-THEIR-MIND': How Deaf Teachers Select Sign Language Interpreters in Hà Nội, Việt Nam." In *Sign Language Ideologies in Practice*, edited by Annelies Kusters, Mara Green, Erin Moriarty, and Kristin Snoddon, 129–144. Berlin: De Gruyter Mouton; Lancaster, UK: Ishara Press.

Marsilli-Vargas, Xochitl. 2014. "Listening Genres: The Emergence of Relevance Structures through the Reception of Sound." *Journal of Pragmatics*, no. 69: 42–51.

Massey, Doreen. 1994. *Space, Place, and Gender*. Cambridge, UK: Polity Press.

Mathur, Gaurav, and Donna Jo Napoli. 2011. "Introduction: Why Go around the Deaf World?" In *Deaf around the World: The Impact of Language*, edited by Gaurav Mathur and Donna Jo Napoli, 3–15. Oxford, UK: Oxford University Press.

Mauldin, Laura. 2014. "Precarious Plasticity: Neuropolitics, Cochlear Implants, and the Redefinition of Deafness." *Science, Technology, and Human Values* 39 (1): 130–153.

Mauss, Marcel. 1973 [1936]. "Techniques of the Body." *Economy and Society* 2 (1): 70–88.

Mayberry, Rachel I. 2010. "Early Language Acquisition and Adult Language Ability: What Sign Language Reveals about the Critical Period for Language." In *The Oxford Handbook of Deaf Studies, Language, and Education,* volume 2, edited by Marc Marschark and Patricia Elizabeth Spencer, 281–291. New York: Oxford University Press.

McHugh, Ernestine L. 1989. "Concepts of the Person among the Gurungs of Nepal." *American Ethnologist* 16 (1): 75–86.

Meek, Barbra A. 2011. *We Are Our Language: An Ethnography of Language Revitalization in a Northern Athabaskan Community.* Tucson: University of Arizona Press.

Meek, Laura A., and Julia Alejandra Morales Fontanilla. 2022. "Otherwise." *Feminist Anthropology* 3 (2): 274–283.

Meier, Richard P. 1987. "Elicited Imitation of Verb Agreement in American Sign Language: Iconically or Morphologically Determined?" *Journal of Memory and Language* 26 (3): 362–376.

Meir, Irit, Wendy Sandler, Carol Padden, and Mark Aronoff. 2010. "Emerging Sign Languages." In *The Oxford Handbook of Deaf Studies, Language, and Education,* volume 2, edited by Marc Marschark and Patricia Elizabeth Spencer, 267–280. Oxford, UK: Oxford University Press.

Merleau-Ponty, Maurice. 1945 [1967]. *Phénomenologie de la perception.* Paris: Editions Gallimard.

Mills, Mara. 2012. "Do Signals Have Politics? Inscribing Abilities in Cochlear Implants." In *The Oxford Handbook of Sound Studies,* edited by Trevor Pinch and Karin Bijsterveld, 320–346. Oxford, UK: Oxford University Press.

Mitchell, Ross E., and Michaela Karchmer. 2004. "Chasing the Mythical Ten Percent: Parental Hearing Status of Deaf and Hard of Hearing Students in the United States." *Sign Language Studies* 4 (2): 138–163.

Moges, Rezenet. 2018. "The Signs of Deaf Female Masculinity: Styles of Gendering/Queering ASL." In *The Oxford Handbook of Language and Sexuality* (online edition), edited by Kira Hall and Rusty Barrett. Accessed October 12, 2022. https://doi.org/10.1093/oxfordhb/9780190212926.013.64_update_001.

Monaghan, Leila Frances, Karen Nakamura, Constanze Schmaling, and Graham H. Turner, eds. 2003. *Many Ways To Be Deaf: International Variation in Deaf Communities.* Washington, DC: Gallaudet University Press.

Moore, Liz. 2020. "I'm Tired of Chasing a Cure." In *Disability Visibility: First-Person Stories from the Twenty-First Century,* edited by Alice Wong, 75–81. New York: Vintage Books.

Moriarty, Erin. 2019. "Deaf People with 'No Language': Mobility and Flexible Accumulation in Language Practices of Deaf People in Cambodia." *Applied Linguistics Review* 10 (1): 55–72.

Moriarty, Erin, and Lynn Hou. 2023. "Deaf Communities: Constellations, Entanglements, and Defying Classifications." In *A New Companion to Linguistic Anthropology,* edited by Alessandro Duranti, Rachel George, and Robin Conley Riner, 122–138. Hoboken, NJ: John Wiley and Sons.

Moriarty, Erin, and Annelies Kusters. 2021. "Deaf Cosmopolitanism: Calibrating as a Moral Process." *International Journal of Multilingualism* 18 (2): 285–302.

Nagai, Julia, and Edwin K. Everhart. 2022. "Oral English Proficiency Tests, Interpretive Labor, and the Neoliberal University." *Journal of Linguistic Anthropology* 32 (3): 543–560. https://doi.org/10.1111/jola.12374.

Napier, Jemina. 2021. *Sign Language Brokering in Deaf-Hearing Families*. Cham, UK: Palgrave Macmillan.

Narayan, Kirin. 2002. "Placing Lives through Stories: Second-Generation South Asian Americans." In *Everyday Life in South Asia*, edited by Diane Minesa and Sarah Lamb, 425–39. Bloomington: Indiana University Press.

National Federation of the Deaf Nepal (NDFN). 2003. *Nepāli Sānketik Bhāshāko Shabda-kosh (Nepali Sign Language Dictionary)*. Kathmandu: Nepal National Federation of the Deaf and Hard of Hearing.

Neveu, Grace. 2020. "When Deafness Is Not Considered a Deficit." *Sapiens*. Accessed September 30, 2022. https://medium.com/sapiens-org/when-deafness-is-not-considered-a-deficit-82fd4521b128.

———. 2019. "Lexical Conventionalization and the Emergence of Grammatical Devices in a Second Generation Homesign System in Peru." PhD dissertation. University of Texas–Austin.

Nguyen, Xuan Thuy. 2018. "Critical Disability Studies at the Edge of Global Development: Why Do We Need to Engage with Southern Theory?." *Canadian Journal of Disability Studies* 7 (1): 1–25. https://doi.org/10.15353/cjds.v7i1.400.

Nonaka, Angela M. 2012. "Language Ecological Change in Ban Khor, Thailand: An Ethnographic Case Study of Village Sign Language Endangerment." In *Sign Languages in Village Communities: Anthropological and Linguistic Insights*, edited by Ulrike Zeshan and Connie de Vos, 277–312. Berlin: Walter de Gruyter; Nijmegen: Ishara Press.

———. 2009. "Estimating Size, Scope, and Membership of the Speech/Sign Communities of Undocumented Indigenous/Village Sign Languages: The Ban Khor Case Study." *Language and Communication* 29: 210–229.

———. 2007. "Emergence of an Indigenous Sign Language and a Speech/Sign Community in Ban Khor, Thailand." PhD dissertation. University of California, Los Angeles.

Nyst, Victoria. 2012. "Shared Sign Languages." In *Sign Language: An International Handbook*, edited by Roland Pfau, M. Steinbach, and Bencie Woll, 552–574. Berlin: Mouton de Gruyter.

Nyst, Victoria, Kara Sylla, and Moustapha Magassouba. 2012. "Deaf Signers in Douentza, a Rural Area in Mali." In *Sign Languages in Village Communities: Anthropological and Linguistic Insights*, edited by Ulrike Zeshan and Connie de Vos, 251–276. Berlin: Walter de Gruyter; Nijmegen: Ishara Press.

Padden, Carol. 1981. "Some Arguments for Syntactic Patterning in American Sign Language." *Sign Language Studies*, no. 32: 239–259.

Padden, Carol, and Tom Humphries. 1988. *Deaf in America: Voices from a Culture*. Cambridge, MA: Harvard University Press.

Padden, Carol, So-One Hwang, Ryan Lepic, and Aron Seegers. 2015. "Tools for Language: Patterned Iconicity in Sign Language Nouns and Verbs." *Topics in Cognitive Science* 7 (1): 81–94.

Padden, Carol A. 2011. "Sign Language Geography." In *Deaf around the World: The Impact of Language*, edited by Gaurav Mathur and Donna Jo Napoli, 19–37. Oxford: Oxford University Press.

Padden, Carol A., and David M. Perlmutter. 1987. "American Sign Language and the Architecture of Phonological Theory." *Natural Language and Linguistic Theory* 5 (3): 335–375.

Padden, Carol A., Irit Meir, So-One Hwang, Ryan Lepic, Aron Seegers, and Tory Sampson. 2013. "Patterned Iconicity in Sign Language Lexicons." *Gesture* 13 (3): 287–308.

Panda, Sibaji. 2012. "A Sociolinguistic and Cultural Profile." In *Sign Languages in Village Communities: Anthropological and Linguistic Insights*, edited by Ulrike Zeshan and Connie de Vos, 353–360. Berlin: Walter de Gruyter; Nijmegen: Ishara Press.

Pandian, Anand, and Daud Ali, eds. 2010. *Ethical Life in South Asia*. Bloomington: Indiana University Press.

Peirce, Charles. 1955. "Logic as Semiotic." In *Philosophical Writings of Peirce*, edited by Justus Buchler, 98–155. New York: Dover Publications.

Perniss, Pamela, and Gabriella Vigliocco. 2014. "The Bridge of Iconicity: From a World of Experience to the Experience of Language." *Philosophical Transactions of the Royal Society B: Biological Sciences* 369 (1651): 20130300.

Perniss, Pamela, Robin L. Thompson, and Gabriella Vigliocco. 2010. "Iconicity as a General Property of Language: Evidence from Spoken and Signed Languages." *Frontiers in Psychology* 1, article 227.

Piepzna-Samarasinha, Leah Lakshmi. 2022. *The Future is Disabled: Prophecies, Love Notes, and Mourning Songs*. Vancouver, BC: Arsenal Pulp Press.

Pigg, Stacey Leigh. 1996. "The Credible and the Credulous: The Question of "Villagers' Beliefs" in Nepal." *Cultural Anthropology* 11 (2): 160–201.

———. 1992. "Inventing Social Categories through Place: Social Representations and Development in Nepal." *Comparative Studies in Society and History* 34 (3): 491–513.

Pizzuto, Elena, and Virginia Volterra. 2000. "Iconicity and Transparency in Sign Languages: A Cross-Linguistic Cross-Cultural View." In *The Signs of Language Revisited: An Anthology to Honor Ursula Bellugi and Edward Klima*, edited by Karen Emmorey and Harlan Lane, 261–286. Mahwah, NJ: Lawrence Erlbaum Associates Publishers.

Povinelli, Elizabeth. 2011. "Routes/Worlds." *E-flux* 27 (September). Accessed September 29, 2022. www.e-flux.com/journal/27/67991/routes-worlds.

———. 2002. *The Cunning of Recognition: Indigenous Alterities and the Making of Australian Multiculturalism*. Durham, NC: Duke University Press.

Pradhan, Uma. 2020. *Simultaneous Identities: Language, Education, and the Nepali Nation*. Cambridge, UK: Cambridge University Press.

Prasad, Lakshmi Narayan. 2003. *Status of People with Disability (People with Different Ability) in Nepal*. Kathmandu: Rajesh Prasad Shrivastav.

Prasad, Leela. 2010. "Ethical Subjects: Time, Telling, and Tellability." In *Ethical Life in South Asia*, edited by Anand Pandian and Daud Ali, 174–191. Bloomington: Indiana University Press.

Reed, Lauren W. 2022. "Sign Networks: Nucleated Network Sign Languages and Rural Homesign in Papua New Guinea." *Language in Society* 51 (4): 627–661.

———. 2020. "'Switching Caps': Two Ways of Communicating in Sign in the Port Moresby Deaf Community, Papua New Guinea." *Asia-Pacific Language Variation* 6 (1): 13–52.

Reed, Lauren, Alan Rumsey, Francesca Merlan, and John Onga. 2018. "The Communicative Ecology of Deaf Sign Languages in the Western Highlands of Papua New Guinea: A Powerpoint Seminar Presentation with Embedded Video." Accessed on February 23, 2021. www.academia.edu/37934872/The_communicative_ecology_of_deaf_sign_languages _in_the_Western_Highlands_of_Papua_New_Guinea_A_Powerpoint_seminar_pre sentation_with_embedded_video.

Reno, Joshua. 2012. "Technically Speaking: On Equipping and Evaluating 'Unnatural' Language Learners." *American Anthropologist* 114 (3): 406–419.

Restrepo, Eduardo, and Arturo Escobar. 2005. "'Other Anthropologies and Anthropology Otherwise': Steps to a World Anthropologies Framework." *Critique of Anthropology* 25 (2): 99–129.

Rhodes, Catherine R. 2020. "Dually Authenticated and Doubly Modern: Institutionalizing Jach Maaya in the Yucatan Today." *Journal of Linguistic Anthropology* 30 (3): 326–352.

Rickford, John R., and Sharese King. 2016. "Language and Linguistics on Trial: Hearing Rachel Jeantel (and Other Vernacular Speakers) in the Courtroom and Beyond." *Language*: 948–988.

Robinson, Kelly Fagan. 2022. "Knowing by DEAF-Listening: Epistemologies and Ontologies Revealed in Song-Signing." *American Anthropologist* 124 (4): 866–879.

Rosenthal, Abigal. 2009. "Lost in Transcription: The Problematics of Commensurability in Academic Representations of American Sign Language." *Text and Talk: An Interdisciplinary Journal of Language, Discourse and Communication Studies* 29 (5): 595–614.

Rumsey, Alan. 2010. "Ethics, Language, and Human Sociality." In *Ordinary Ethics: Anthropology, Language, and Action*, edited by Michael Lambek, 105–122. New York: Fordham University Press.

Rutherford, Danilyn. 2021. "Becoming an Operating System: Disability, Difference, and the Ethics of Communication in the United States." *American Ethnologist* 48 (2): 139–152.

Sanchez, Rebecca. 2020. "Deafness and Sound." In *Cambridge Critical Concepts: Literature and Sound*, edited by Anna Snaith, 272–286. Cambridge, UK: Cambridge University Press.

Sandler, Wendy. 2012. "Dedicated Gestures and the Emergence of Sign Language." *Gesture* 12 (3): 265–307.

Sarajevo Times. 2013. "Deaf People Gathered Outside B&H Parliament Today To Demand End to Discrimination." Accessed August 17, 2023. https://sarajevotimes.com/deaf-people-gathered-outside-bh-parliament-today-to-demand-end-to-discrimination/.

Saussure, Ferdinand de. 1972. *Course in General Linguistics.* Translated by Roy Harris. Edited by Charles Bally, Albert Sechehaye, and Albert Riedlinger. Chicago: Open Court.

Savolainen, Ulla. 2017. "Tellability, Frame and Silence: The Emergence of Internment Memory." *Narrative Inquiry* 27 (1): 24–46.

Schmidt, Ruth Laila. 1994 [1993]. *A Practical Dictionary of Modern Nepali.* Delhi: Ratna Sagar. Accessed May 30, 2014. http://dsal.uchicago.edu/dictionaries/schmidt/.

Schutz, Alfred. 1970. *On Phenomenology and Social Relations.* Edited by Helmut R. Wagner. Chicago: University of Chicago Press.

Sehyr, Zed Sevcikova, and Karen Emmorey. 2019. "The Perceived Mapping between Form and Meaning in American Sign Language Depends on Linguistic Knowledge and Task: Evidence from Iconicity and Transparency Judgments." *Language and Cognition* 11 (2): 208–234.

Senghas, Richard. 2003. "New Ways To Be Deaf in Nicaragua: Changes in Language, Personhood, and Community." In *Many Ways to be Deaf: International Variation in Deaf Communities*, edited by Leila Frances Monaghan, Karen Nakamura, Constanze Schmaling, and Graham H. Turner, 260–282. Washington, DC: Gallaudet University Press.

Sequenzia, Amy, and Elizabeth J. Grace, eds. 2015. *Typed Words, Loud Voices.* Fort Worth, TX: Autonomous Press, 2015.

Sharma, Shilu. 2003. "The Origin and Development of Nepali Sign Language." MA thesis. Tribhuvan University, Kathmandu.

Shuman, Malcolm K. 1980. "The Sound of Silence in Nohya: A Preliminary Account of Sign Language Use by the Deaf in a Maya Community in Yucatan, Mexico." *Language Sciences* 2 (1): 144–173.

Sidnell, Jack. 2010. "The Ordinary Ethics of Everyday Talk." In *Ordinary Ethics: Anthropology, Language, and Action*, edited by Michael Lambek, 123–139. New York: Fordham University Press.

Silverstein, Michael. 1976. "Shifters, Verbal Categories, and Cultural Description." In *Meaning in Anthropology*, edited by Keith Basso and Henry Selby, 11–55. Albuquerque, NM: School of American Research.

Simpson, Audra. 2014. *Mohawk Interruptus: Political Life across the Borders of Settler States.* Durham, NC: Duke University Press.

Singh, Harischandra Lal. 2004. *Students' Companion Dictionary: English-Nepali, Nepali-English.* Kathmandu: Educational Publishing House.

Sirvage, Robert. 2015. "Measuring the Immeasurable: The Legacy of Atomization and Dorsality as a Pathway in Making Deaf Epistemology Quantifiable—An Insight from DeafSpace." TEDxGallaudet Lecture in American Sign Language. Accessed September 16, 2022. www.youtube.com/watch?v=EPTrOO6EYCY. English translation approved by Robert Sirvage, translated and shared by Terra Edwards.

Slobin, Dan I. 2008. "Breaking the Molds: Signed Languages and the Nature of Human Language." *Sign Language Studies* 8 (2): 114–130.

Snoddon, Kristin. 2022. "Writing as Being: On the Existential Primacy of Writing for a Deaf Scholar." *Qualitative Inquiry* 28 (6): 722–731.

———. 2019. *Report on Baseline Data Collection on Deaf Education in Nepal.* World Federation of the Deaf. Accessed August 16, 2023. http://wfdeaf.org/news/resources/report-baseline-data-collection-deaf-education-nepal/.

Snoddon, Kristin, and Krishna Madaparthi. 2022. "Conceptualizing the Role of Mediation in an Online American Sign Language Teaching Model for Hearing Parents of Deaf Children." *Deafness and Education International* 25 (1): 4–20.

Soldatic, Karen, and Shaun Grech. 2014. "Transnationalising Disability Studies: Rights, Justice and Impairment." *Disability Studies Quarterly* 34 (2). Accessed August 17, 2023. https://dsq-sds.org/index.php/dsq/article/view/4249/3588.

Stokoe, William. 1960. *Sign Language Structure: An Outline of the Visual Communication Systems of the American Deaf.* Buffalo, NY: Department of Anthropology and Linguistics, University oof Buffalo.

Taub, Sarah F. 2001. *Language from the Body: Iconicity and Metaphor in American Sign Language.* Cambridge, UK: Cambridge University Press.

Taverniers, Miriam. 2006. "Grammatical Metaphor and Lexical Metaphor: Different Perspectives on Semantic Variation." *Neophilologus* 90 (2): 321–332.

Taylor, Charles. 1994. *Multiculturalism: Examining the Politics of Recognition.* Princeton, NJ: Princeton University Press.

Taylor, Irene. 1997. *Buddhas in Disguise: Deaf People in Nepal.* San Diego: Dawn Sign Press.

Thompson, Robin L. 2011. "Iconicity in Language Processing and Acquisition: What Signed Languages Reveal." *Language and Linguistics Compass* 5 (9): 603–616.

Torigoe, Takashi, and Wataru Takei. 2002. "A Descriptive Analysis of Pointing and Oral Movements in a Home Sign System." *Sign Language Studies* 2 (3): 281–295.

Torigoe, Takashi, Wataru Takei, and Harumi Kimura. 1995. "Deaf Life on Isolated Japanese Islands." *Sign Language Studies* 87 (Summer): 67–174.

Trawick, Margaret. 1990. *Notes on Love in a Tamil Family*. Berkeley: University of California Press.

Turin, Mark. 2014. "Mother Tongues and Language Competence: The Shifting Politics of Linguistic Belonging in the Himalayas." In *Facing Globalization in the Himalayas: Belonging and the Politics of the Self*, edited by Gérard Toffin and Joanna Pfaff-Czarnecka, 372–396. New Delhi: Sage Publications.

———. 2002. "Call Me Uncle: An Outsider's Experience of Nepali Kinship." *Contributions to Nepalese Studies* 28 (2): 277–283.

United Nations (UN). 2006. *Convention on the Rights of People with Disabilities*. Accessed August 17, 2003. https://social.desa.un.org/issues/disability/crpd/convention-on-the -rights-of-persons-with-disabilities-crpd.

Veditz, George. 1912. "President's Message." In *Proceedings of the Ninth Convention of the National Association of the Deaf and the Third World's Congress of the Deaf, 1910*. Philadelphia, PA: Philocophus Press.

Venkat, Bharat Jayram. 2021. *At the Limits of Cure*. Durham, NC: Duke University Press.

———. 2017. "Scenes of Commitment." *Cultural Anthropology* 32 (1): 93–116.

Washabaugh, William. 1980a. "The Manu-Facturing of a Language." *Sign Language Studies*, no. 29: 291–330.

———. 1980b. "The Organization and Use of Providence Island Sign Language." *Sign Language Studies*, no. 26: 65–92.

Washabaugh, William, James Woodward, and Susan DeSantis. 1978. "Providence Island Sign: A Context-Dependent Language." *Anthropological Linguistics* 20 (3): 95–109.

Weber, Max. 1947. "Social Action and Its Types." In *Theories of Society: Foundations of Modern Sociological Theory*, edited by Talcott Parsons, Edward Shils, Kaspar D. Naegele, and Jesse R. Pitts, 173–179. 1961; New York: Free Press of Glencoe.

Weinberg, Miranda. 2018. "Schooling Languages: Indigeneity, Language Policy and Language Shift in Nepal." PhD dissertation, University of Pennsylvania.

Wilcox, Sherman. 2004. "Hands and Bodies, Minds and Souls: What Can Signed Languages Tell Us About the Origin of Signs?" In *In The Beginning: Origins of Semiosis*, edited by M. Alac and P. Violi, 137–167. Turnhout, Belgium: Brepols.

Woodward, James. 2000. "Sign Languages and Sign Language Families in Thailand and Vietnam." In *The Signs of Language Revisited: An Anthology to Honor Ursula Bellugi and Edward Klima*, edited by Karen Emmorey and Harlan L. Lane, 23–47. New York: Psychology Press.

World Federation of the Deaf (WFD). 2010. "21st International Congress on the Education of the Deaf (ICED) in July 2010 in Vancouver, Canada." Accessed September 6, 2023. https://wfdeaf.org/news/21st-international-congress-on-the-education-of-the-deaf -iced-in-july-2010-in-vancouver-canada/.

Yergeau, M. Remi. 2018. *Authoring Autism: On Rhetoric and Neurological Queerness*. Durham, NC: Duke University Press.

Zeshan, Ulrike. 2011. "Village Sign Languages: A Commentary." In *Deaf around the World: The Impact of Language*, edited by Gaurav Mathur and Donna Jo Napoli, 221–230. Oxford, UK: Oxford University Press.

INDEX

Founded in 1893,
UNIVERSITY OF CALIFORNIA PRESS
publishes bold, progressive books and journals
on topics in the arts, humanities, social sciences,
and natural sciences—with a focus on social
justice issues—that inspire thought and action
among readers worldwide.

The UC PRESS FOUNDATION
raises funds to uphold the press's vital role
as an independent, nonprofit publisher, and
receives philanthropic support from a wide
range of individuals and institutions—and from
committed readers like you. To learn more, visit
ucpress.edu/supportus.